Register Now for Online Access to Your Book!

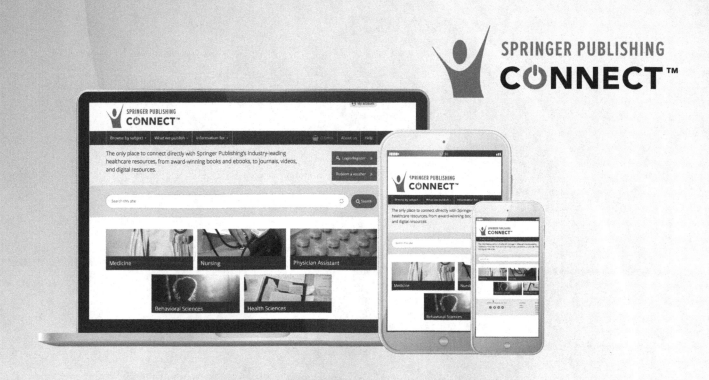

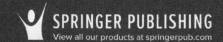

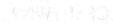

101 PRIMARY CARE CASE STUDIES

Sampath ("Sam") Wijesinghe, DHSc, PA-C, AAHIVS, is a principal faculty member and clinical site director for the Central Valley California region at Stanford University School of Medicine's master's in science physician assistant program. He completed his PA education at Union College, where he received a master's degree in PA studies. He also has a master's degree in management information systems from the University of Nebraska and a doctor of health science degree with an emphasis in global health from A.T. Still University. Dr. Wijesinghe completed an HIV and AIDS clinical fellowship at University of California San Francisco, Fresno. He has been an HIV/AIDS specialist since 2014 and has worked in primary care medicine since 2010, primarily in underserved communities. He has been involved in medical education since 2013. His clinical interests include primary care medicine, HIV medicine, and global health.

Prior to joining Stanford University School of Medicine, Dr. Wijesinghe was a clinical assistant professor at University of California, Davis. Dr. Wijesinghe practices primary care medicine and HIV medicine at Adventist Health Medical Center, Fowler, a small town in California, and Madera Community Hospital in Madera, California.

Dr. Wijesinghe is passionate about teaching the next generation of clinicians. He has practiced in areas of need, including primary care and HIV medicine in underserved areas. He is passionate about medical education because it is an opportunity to improve patient outcomes and give back to the profession. A highly sought-after speaker and lecturer, Dr. Wijesinghe has presented at several national conferences and events and educates the next generation of PAs as a clinical preceptor.

Dr. Wijesinghe lives with his wife, Nuwan, and has two children, Rynee and Ryler. He loves to travel with his family, listen to music, watch sports, and play sports whenever possible.

101 PRIMARY CARE CASE STUDIES

A Workbook for Clinical and Bedside Skills

Sampath Wijesinghe, DHSc, MS, MPAS, AAHIVS, PA-C
Editor/Author

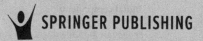

Copyright © 2021 Springer Publishing Company, LLC

Springer Publishing Company, LLC
11 West 42nd Street, New York, NY 10036
www.springerpub.com
connect.springerpub.com/

Acquisitions Editor: Suzanne Toppy
Compositor: diacriTech

ISBN: 9780826182722
ebook ISBN: 9780826182739
DOI: 10.1891/9780826182739

21 22 23 24 / 5 4 3 2 1

The author and the publisher of this Work have made every effort to use sources believed to be reliable to provide information that is accurate and compatible with the standards generally accepted at the time of publication. Because medical science is continually advancing, our knowledge base continues to expand. Therefore, as new information becomes available, changes in procedures become necessary. We recommend that the reader always consult current research and specific institutional policies before performing any clinical procedure or delivering any medication. The author and publisher shall not be liable for any special, consequential, or exemplary damages resulting, in whole or in part, from the readers' use of, or reliance on, the information contained in this book. The publisher has no responsibility for the persistence or accuracy of URLs for external or third-party Internet websites referred to in this publication and does not guarantee that any content on such websites is, or will remain, accurate or appropriate.

Library of Congress Control Number: 2020914270

Contact sales@springerpub.com to receive discount rates on bulk purchases.

Publisher's Note: New and used products purchased from third-party sellers are not guaranteed for quality, authenticity, or access to any included digital components.

Printed in the United States of America.

This book is dedicated to

My mentor, Alex Moir (1962–2015), who taught me true compassion and was a mentor and role model beyond compare. It was always my dream that we'd coauthor this book, but that dream could not come true. The world lost a fine man, who could have taught compassion and competent care to generations of future clinicians.

My parents, David (1944–2015) and Rita Wijesinghe. When I was growing up, our family did not have much, but my parents' unconditional love and fight to provide a better future for me and my loving sister Mangali laid a solid foundation for our journeys. Importantly, my parents always believed in me. I love you more!

My wife, Nuwan. Meeting you in high school was the best thing that ever happened to me. Marrying you was the best decision I ever made. Everything I do personally or professionally is possible because you are in my life. I love you more than you can imagine.

My children, Rynee and Ryler. Throughout the preparation of this book, you both selflessly gave me the space and time I needed. I know I have taken too much time away from you because of this publication. Your love and support from the beginning to end has meant the world to me. You two are the reason I want to contribute and make the world a better place!

PAs, NPs, physicians, and future clinicians. We know practicing medicine and lifelong learning are inseparable. Let's continue to support each other and learn from one another. I applaud your decision to practice medicine and make a difference in many people's lives.

CONTENTS

CONTRIBUTORS

Valerie Berry, MD
Assistant Professor
Master of Science Physician Assistant Program
College of Health Sciences and Human Services
California State University, Monterey Bay
Salinas, California

Michael S. Burney, EdD, MS, PA-C
Program Director/Chair, Clinical Associate
Professor
Chapman University PA Program
Crean College of Health and Behavioral Sciences
Irvine, California

Michael Castillo, MD
Department of Family Medicine
Kaiser Permanente
Fresno, California

Rachel Chappell, MHSc, PA-C
Program Director, Clinical Assistant Professor
Interdisciplinary Human Studies, Physician
Assistant Program
School of Allied Health Professions
Louisiana State University Health Science Center
New Orleans, Louisiana

Mark P. Christiansen, PhD, PA-C
Program Director and Department Chair
Physician Assistant Program
Department of Physician Assistant Education
University of the Pacific
Sacramento, California

Dolores Davis, RN, FNP APRN-C
Madera Community Hospital, Family Health
Services
VA Central California Health Care System
Fresno, California

David Duensing, DO
Pediatrics, PC
Lincoln, NE
University of Nebraska Medical Center
Adjunct Associate Professor
Department of Pediatrics
Omaha, Nebraska

Volunteer Clinical Preceptor, Advanced Practice
Nursing Program
University of Nebraska Medical Center
Omaha, Nebraska
Volunteer Clinical Preceptor, Physician Assistant
Program
Union College
Lincoln, Nebraska

Christopher P. Forest, DHSc, DFAAPA, PA-C
Founding PA Program Director
Master of Science Physician Assistant Program
College of Health Sciences and Human Services
California State University, Monterey Bay
Salinas, California

Tosi Gilford, MD, PA-C
Program Director, Assistant Professor
Physician Assistant Studies Program, Clinical and
Diagnostic Sciences Department
University of Alabama at Birmingham
Birmingham, Alabama

Nancy Hamler, DMSc, MPA, RDN, PA-C
Assistant Professor
Physician Assistant Program
Department of Physician Assistant Education
University of the Pacific
Sacramento, California

Surani Hayre-Kwan, MBA, DNP, FNP-BC, FACHE, FAANP
Director, Professional Practice & Nursing Excellence
Sutter Health
Sacramento, California
Nurse Practitioner, Russian River Health Center
Guerneville, California

Cherilyn M. Hendrix, DHEd, MSBME, PA-C, DFAAPA
Program Director/Associate Professor
University of Maryland Baltimore/Anne Arundel
Community College Collaborative Physician
Assistant Program
University of Maryland Baltimore Graduate School
Baltimore, Maryland

Lisa Hood, DNP, MSN, RN, FNP-C
Family Nurse Practitioner
Family Health Services
Madera Community Hospital
Madera, California

Michael J. Huckabee, PhD, MPAS, PA-C
Director, Physician Assistant Program
Associate Professor, Senior Associate Consultant-II
College of Medicine and Sciences
Mayo Clinic
Rochester, Minnesota

Amanda J. Ingalls, MS, PA-C
Clinical Instructor of Family Medicine
Physician Assistant Program
Keck School of Medicine
University of Southern California
Alhambra, California

Johnny Jimenez, MSN, APRN, FNP-C
Nurse Practitioner, Family Medicine
Sutter Health
Memorial Hospital Los Banos
Los Banos, California

Paramjit Kaur, MSN, FNP-C
Past Family Practice Nurse Practitioner
Adventist Medical Clinic
Sanger, California

Gerald Kayingo, PhD, MMSc, PA-C
Executive Director, Assistant Dean and Professor
Physician Assistant Leadership and Learning
Academy
University of Maryland Graduate School
Baltimore, Maryland

Jason R. Kessler, MD, FAAP
Medical Director/Pediatrician
Primary Health Care, Inc.
Des Moines, Iowa

Vasco Deon Kidd, DHSc, MPH, MS, PA-C
Office of Advanced Practice and UCI
Health Department of Orthopaedic Surgery
Orange, California

Timothy Kuntz, MPAS, PA-C
Assistant Professor
Physician Assistant Program
Union College
Lincoln, Nebraska

Aimee Larson, MSPA, PA-C
Program Director, Clinical Assistant Professor
School of Education and Human Services
Canisius College Physician Assistant Studies
Buffalo, New York

Susan LeLacheur, DrPH, PA-C
Professor of Physician Assistant Studies
The George Washington University School of
Medicine and Health Sciences
Washington, DC

Kristy Luciano, MS, PA-C
Assistant Professor and Director of Didactic Education
Physician Assistant Program
College of Health Sciences
Midwestern University
Downers Grove, Illinois

Erin N. Lunn, PA-C, MHS
Assistant Professor, Director of Clinical Education
Department of Physician Assistant Studies
University of South Alabama
Mobile, Alabama

Hema Majeno, PA-C
Internal Medicine/Hospitalist PA-C
Mercy Hospital
Merced, California

David Malebranche, MD, MPH
Associate Professor of Medicine
Department of Medicine
Morehouse School of Medicine
Atlanta, Georgia

April H. Martin, MSPAS, PA-C
Program Director and Assistant Professor
School of Health Sciences
Francis Marion University
Florence, South Carolina

Mario Martinez, MD
Program Director
Kaweah Delta Family Medicine Residency Program
Visalia, California
Medical Director
Adventist Health Community Care Clinic, Central
Valley Network
Hospitalist, Vituity-Adventist Community Hospital
Reedley, California

Lynn H. McComas, DNP, ANP-C, PHN
President/CEO, PreceptorLink
Encinitas, California

**Kameko Hazley McGuire, DNP, PMHNP-BC,
NP-C, RN**
Visiting Professor, Chamberlain University
MSN-FNP Program
Downers Grove, Illinois
Adjunct Faculty, Regis College PMHNP Program
Weston, Massachusetts
Adjunct Faculty, South University FNP Program
Savannah, Georgia
Graduate Adjunct PMHNP Professor
Liberty University
Lynchburg, Virginia

Jennifer Momen, MD, MPH, FAAP
Assistant Professor, Program Director
Department of Human Performance
Division of Physician Assistant Studies
West Virginia University School of Medicine
Morgantown, West Virginia

Michael N. Moya, MD
Academic Hospitalist
Associate Program Director
Family Medicine Residency Program
Department Chair, Family Medicine
St. Agnes Medical Center
Fresno, California

Andrew Nevins, MD
Clinical Associate Professor
Stanford University School of Medicine
Stanford, California

Karen Paolinelli, MSN, APRN, FNP-C, PA-C, DFAAPA
CEO/President
Madera Community Hospital
Madera, California

Shantha Parameswaran, MD, FAAP
Pediatrician
One Community Health
Sacramento, California

Tushar M. Patel, MD
Pediatrician
Children's Medical Centers of Fresno
Fresno, California

Jason Radke, MMS, PA-C
Department Chair & Program Director
Assistant Professor
College of Health Professions
Rosalind Franklin University of Medicine and Science
North Chicago, Illinois

Jennifer Ramos, MPAP, PA-C
Clinical Instructor of Family Medicine
Physician Assistant Program
Keck School of Medicine
University of Southern California
Alhambra, California

Karla Reinhart DNP, FNP-C, ARNP
Murphy Creek Wellness, Nurse Practitioner/Owner
Medford, Oregon
Oregon Health & Science University
Ashland, Oregon

Sara Rygol, MPAS, PA-C
Primary Care Physician Assistant
CHI Health Clinic
Council Bluffs, Iowa

Alfred M. Sadler Jr, MD, FACP, ScD (Hon)
Master of Science Physician Assistant Program
College of Health Sciences and Human Services
California State University, Monterey Bay
Salinas, California

Anabel Segovia, RN, MSN, FNP-C
Nurse Practitioner
Sierra Kings
Reedley, California

Tana Summers, MS, PA-C
Assistant Program Director
Physician Assistant Program
Samuel Merritt University
Oakland, California

Laura L. Van Auker, DNP, APRN, FNP-BC, MSN, SN-C
Assistant Clinical Professor
Betty Irene Moore School of Nursing
University of California, Davis
Sacramento, California

James Van Rhee, MS, PA-C
Program Director/Associate Professor
Yale School of Medicine, Physician Assistant Online Program
Yale University
New Haven, Connecticut

Veronica Vo, MPAC, PA-C
Family Medicine Physician Assistant
Family Healthcare Network
Hanford, California

Anne Walsh, PA-C, MMSc, DFAAPA
Clinical Associate Professor
Chapman University PA Program
Crean College of Health and Behavioral Sciences
Irvine, California

Ariel L. Watriss, MSN, NP-C
Nurse Practitioner, Sexual Health Specialist
College of Health Nurse Practitioner
Tufts University Health Services
Medford, Massachusetts

Jennifer C. Weeks, DNP, FNP-C
Family Nurse Practitioner
MedNow Urgent and Primary Care
Augusta, Georgia

Sampath Wijesinghe, DHSc, PA-C, AAHIVS
Principal Faculty, Master of Science in Physician Assistant Studies
Stanford School of Medicine
Primary Care PA-C and HIV Specialist
at Adventist Health
Central Valley Network, California
Primary Care PA-C and HIV Specialist at Madera Community Hospital
Madera, California

REVIEWERS

Krishan Ariyarathna, MD
Internal/Hospital Medicine
Nebraska Hospitalist, LLC
Omaha, Nebraska

Alan Brokenicky, MPAS, PA-C
Academic Co-Director
Physician Assistant Studies Program
College of Medicine and Sciences
Mayo Clinic
Rochester, Minnesota

Joan Caruso, MPAS, PA-C
Physician Assistant Program Director/Chair,
Clinical Assistant Professor
Department of Physician Assistant Studies
Clarkson University
Potsdam, New York

Rachel Chappell, MHSc, PA-C
Program Director, Clinical Assistant Professor
Interdisciplinary Human Studies, Physician
Assistant Program
School of Allied Health Professions
Louisiana State University Health Science Center
New Orleans, Louisiana

Simerjit Singh Dhaliwal, PA-C, MS, RCP
Family Medicine, United Health Centers of
San Joaquin Valley
Selma, California

Christy Eskes, DHSc, MPA, PA-C
Instructor, Former Assistant Professor and Past
Program Director
Department of Physician Assistant Sciences
Loma Linda University
Loma Linda, California
Lead Advanced Practice Provider for Correctional Health
Emergent Medical Associates
Los Angeles, California

Michael Estrada, DHSc, MS, PA-C
Founding Director and Chair
Physician Assistant Program
College of Arts and Sciences
University of La Verne
La Verne, California

Susan M. Fernandes, LPD, PA-C
Associate Dean for PA Education
Clinical Professor of Pediatrics and Medicine
Stanford School of Medicine
Stanford, California

Nichole A. Flores, BA, MA. MAOB, PsyD
Director of Behavioral Health
Behavioral Health, Valley Health Team, Inc.
Kerman, California

Jordan Hairr, EdD, MSPAS, PA-C
Associate Dean
School of Allied Health Professions
Program Director
Department of PA Medicine
Greer, South Carolina

Virginia McCoy Hass, RN, DNP, FNP-C, PA-C
Associate Clinical Professor (retired)
Betty Irene Moore School of Nursing
University of California, Davis
Sacramento, California

Megan Heidtbrink, MPAS, PA-C
Program Director, Associate Professor
Union College Physician Assistant Program
Union College
Lincoln, Nebraska

Cherilyn M. Hendrix, DHEd, MSBME, PA-C, DFAAPA
Program Director/Associate Professor
University of Maryland Baltimore/Anne Arundel
Community College Collaborative Physician
Assistant Program
University of Maryland Baltimore Graduate School
Baltimore, Maryland

Trenton Honda, PhD, MMS, PA-C
Associate Professor and Division Chief
Division of PA Studies
University of Utah
Salt Lake City, Utah

Amanda J. Ingalls, MS, PA-C
Clinical Instructor of Family Medicine
Department of Family Medicine
Division of Physician Assistant Studies
University of Southern California
Alhambra, California

FOREWORD

This is a remarkable collection of primary care case studies, presented in a unique and comprehensive manner. Included is a broad spectrum of cases that emphasize the scientific as well as the psychologic and emotional dimensions of care. We can all learn from each other as physicians, physician assistants, and nurse practitioners. Anyone interested in primary care will benefit from this book.

The book is arranged so you can pick and choose what interests you or relates to a specific case that you have. It is an ideal volume for those engaged in the primary care education of physicians, physician assistants, and nurse practitioners. It will also be a valuable resource for the primary care practitioner.

Besides the standard presentation of a patient problem, each case includes evidence-based information, references for additional reading, ICD-10 and CPT codes (very practical), topics for education, legal concerns, and specific items to be addressed by the broader healthcare team from receptionist to specialist. Bedside manner questions allow the educator or practitioner to expand the scope of inquiry, as time and interest permit. Finally, the narrative by the primary care provider brings the discussion from the didactic/scientific to the personal. I am not aware of any other volume that does this.

I congratulate Sampath Wijesinghe, who is a sterling example of a primary care educator and practitioner, for putting together this remarkable collection of cases and the stories that go with them. I know that the reader will find this multiauthored book invaluable and inspiring.

Alfred M. Sadler Jr MD, FACP, ScD (Hon)
Senior Advisor, California State University
Master of Science Physician Assistant Program,
Salinas, California

FOREWORD

Primary care medicine is the heart of medicine. It is a field where you never know what patient is going to walk through your door next. Frequently, what is listed on the schedule is not what you discover as you sit across from your patient and ask, "So what brings you in today?" It's also not what you discover when you dig a little deeper into a patient's story. More than once, I have called out to my puzzled medical assistant, *"Can you grab me an anoscope?"* for a patient who came in for a sore throat! Variety is part of what makes primary care so wonderful. As a clinician, you also get to build wonderful, long-term relationships, and this is my favorite part of primary care medicine. When you have seen patients year upon year, possibly even from birth, you really get to know them. In time, you recognize when there is a change in the way Mr. Jones is dressed or note that his smile is a little less bright or his steps a little more shuffled. There will likely be a day when your patient says *"You saved my life"* and rewards you with their homemade chocolates. There is never a dull day in primary care medicine, and as clinicians, we really make a difference in the population in which we serve. For these reasons, I love primary care medicine and there is no place I would rather work as a nurse practitioner.

As a new clinician, you will really find it is true when that medicine is both art and science. You will develop your individual approach to the art of medicine. As you learn and grow, you will learn how to master your "medical paintbrush." You will see 10 clinicians might treat the same patient in 10 different ways, and all of them may be correct in their approaches. Listening carefully, *really listening* to a patient, a family, caregivers, will improve your diagnostic skills. You will also learn how to most effectively and thoughtfully deliver education or bad news. Your clinical skills are absolutely vital, but your "soft skills" are invaluable. However, traditional classroom is not the most effective place to learn them. Soft skills come with time and experience and include communication skills, listening skills, and an ability to demonstrate empathy. It is your ability to "read" others. It is a vital part of our skill set as clinicians.

It is our job to earn our patients' trust and to give them the very best care. Even when our schedules are packed with back-to-back appointments and our inbox is stacked with labs and reports to be reviewed, we must remember that "the patient in Room 1" is more than just a CPT code. If primary care medicine is the heart of medicine, then our patients are its soul. We have to work collaboratively as a team—from the front office person, to the clinician, to the biller. We have to treat patients the way we would want to be treated, because some day you may be the patient.

Clinical rotations can be an overwhelming experience for any student. Despite all of your didactic preparation, you may feel completely underprepared. The first year as a new clinician is a formidable learning trajectory. Suddenly, you are making life and death decisions about *your patient. Apps and reference manuals are helpful, but what you really want is real-world advice from those in the trenches, and that is exactly what this book provides. It is a real-world, practical handbook of genuine scenarios. All the cases in the book are real-life case studies shared by the authors. Through a stepwise process, you will be challenged to critically think through the steps of clinical decision-making—from the chief complaint to billing and coding, they are all discussed. In addition to clinical decisions, you will hear each author's approach and some of the soft skills used. This book will be an invaluable asset, not only to a student or new clinician working in primary care but also to the seasoned professional who wants to gain insight by looking at other approaches in the art and science of medicine.*

Lynn H. McComas, DNP, ANP-C, PHN
President/CEO PreceptorLink, Encinitas, California

FOREWORD

Some might say there are plenty of primary care textbooks today. Why one more? I'm here to offer three reasons for *101 Primary Care Case Studies*: the art, the appeal, and the author.

This text reminds us of *the art* of medicine, beyond the requirement to practice by evidence-based medicine. Yes, each case study provides the science and relevant practice guidelines behind a particular and vital diagnosis. To practice medicine solely by evidence alone leads to a risk of recipe-card decisions rather than personalized patient care. Heuristics, when conjoined with evidence, leads to best practice. *101 Primary Care Case Studies* enhances this foundational evidence-based content, integrating the artistic touch of medicine by personalizing each case to a real patient. Each chapter includes the unique section, titled Insight from the PCP, which offers a clinician's pearls of wisdom about bedside manner and achieving optimal patient outcomes based on science and first-hand experience. The book's collection of pearls alone offers tremendous value to the reader seeking to guide patients toward the best health outcomes.

As it is written for primary care providers, this text emphasizes *the appeal* our career offers. In primary care, we have the privilege to develop patient relationships that extend across the lifespan. Representing these cradle-to-grave lives, the case studies in this book read as stories from the family. Only primary care expects a consistent patient relationship that celebrates births, school events, sporting achievements, graduations, marriages, promotions, relocations, retirements, and bereavements, with all the successes and disappointments along the journey. Clinical decisions wrestled in these pages are made with consideration of how it affects the individual life of a patient at a particular time. By reading only a handful of case studies herein, one comes away with how each patient deserves an individualized approach via team-based care with full consideration of the person's current life circumstances. That approach epitomizes why we in primary care love what we do.

Finally, to those who might say we have enough primary care textbooks, you don't know *the author*, Dr. Wijesinghe. He cares for his patients with both exceptional clinical skills and compassionate bedside manners—and emphasizes the importance of both to be a good clinician. He respects all members of the healthcare team as critical to optimal patient care, including receptionists, the cleaning crew, and the ever-important medical assistant. Dr. Wijesinghe seeks to be a part of the solution whenever possible (why he chose primary care medicine in rural clinics including HIV medicine, where healthcare professional shortages are the greatest). So, when using a textbook by an author with this indomitable spirit of integrity, the reader can expect an excellent opportunity to learn from a master among the most caring and professional of clinicians.

For learners entering the primary care professions of health delivery, or for learners with years of medical experience, your library is incomplete without this book. Nothing else combines the art of medicine with the appeal of primary care than what this author has created. We will serve our patients with better care by integrating the pearls of this text into our practices.

Michael J. Huckabee, PhD, MPAS, PA-C
Director, Physician Assistant Program, Associate Professor, Senior Associate Consultant-II,
Mayo Clinic, Rochester, Minnesota

PREFACE

INTRODUCTION

Primary care medicine is the largest medical specialty in the United States. While physician assistants, nurse practitioners, and physicians branch into specialties, a majority practices in primary care. When practicing primary care medicine, clinical skills and soft, or bedside manner, skills are important. Although there are many clinical medicine textbooks for students to learn all the important data about the hundreds of conditions a primary care provider will treat, there are few that use case studies as a primary means to help students work through a real patient scenario to strengthen clinical skills, let alone soft skills, which are often overlooked in a packed clinical curriculum. Current case study products typically focus solely on diagnostic skill. None focus on the combination of both clinical and bedside skills.

This book is intended to bridge the gap between the objective clinical content presented in the didactic phase of a PA, NP, or medical curriculum and the clinical application/rotation phase. It can be used during both phases of a program. Students will use book knowledge to work through a real-life chief complaint presented by a patient, and through a series of questions determine the appropriate focused exam, workup, diagnosis, and treatment for the patient.

Real-life medicine is not organized by organ system or diagnosis. Most often, patients will present with vague descriptions of symptoms, and a PCP will have to surmise the best approach to the problem. For example, a patient who presents with chest pain may have a diagnosis related to the heart, but the problem could also be related to anxiety or reflux.

THE ORIGIN OF THIS BOOK

When I was a PA student, I enjoyed learning from clinicians who shared patient cases. I knew I would see similar cases when I started practice. When I began teaching at the University of California Davis PA/NP program, I taught students based on real cases. I recognized immediately that students are keen to learn from real cases. My experience first as a PA student and then as a medical educator led me to propose a book based on real cases. My initial idea was to write a book to help PA, NP, and medical students acquire competent skills.

MEETING ALEX MOIR

In August 2010, I started practicing primary care medicine in Sanger, a small town in California. I practiced medicine with Dr. Alex Moir, my collaborative physician. During my first week, Dr. Moir invited me to have lunch with him so we could get to know each other. I was looking forward to our lunch and was nervous at the same time. During our lunch, I said, "Dr. Moir, I am happy to work for you." He immediately corrected me, "Please don't think you work for me. I want you to know that you work *with* me. We are one team." On that day, I realized I had the opportunity to work with a great human being. Dr. Moir was my mentor, who practiced competent and compassionate care. I wanted to practice medicine like Dr. Moir practiced medicine. I always thought I was pretty compassionate, but, as I worked with Dr. Moir, I realized my compassionate care skills were developing even more. Dr. Moir was teaching me to deliver compassionate care. I was committed to sharing this powerful message with other clinicians, particularly with future clinicians, by keeping compassionate care central to the book's focus. So, I compiled this book based on real patient cases. I wanted Dr. Alex Moir to coauthor this book, but he died in a tragic accident. My grief put the book on hold for a time.

When I began to think about the book again, I decided I would dedicate it to Dr. Moir, whose mentorship influenced my life as a husband, father, and clinician. With that in mind, I reached out to some PCPs who provide competent and compassionate care to contribute cases. Some have taught me during my didactic training in PA school, some have trained me during my clinical clerkships, some are friends and colleagues, and some are students I had trained. I intentionally included a wide range of experience in this book, from very experienced clinicians to a few new clinicians. I wanted to present a variety of cases from clinicians with short-term and long-term experience. I hope these patient cases help future and practicing clinicians to learn and provide the best care to their patients. This book was a collaborative effort of many people with a common goal: taking care of patients and doing something meaningful for medical education.

The goal of this book is to improve competent skills and bedside skills. There is no disagreement that we can teach competence skills to the next generation and improve clinical skills. However, there is disagreement on whether compassion can be learned. I believe it can be, and there is evidence in support of my belief.

ARE BEDSIDE SKILLS AND COMPASSION NECESSARY?

Compassion is fundamental to the delivery of healthcare,[1] something that patients, families, clinicians, and policy makers all agree.[2] The first principle of the American Medical Education cites compassion as being necessary in the delivery of care.[2] According to the Code of Ethics, "A physician shall be dedicated to providing competent medical care, with compassion and respect for human dignity and rights."[2] PAs and NPs are expected to practice the same. Consequently, compassion is required of all clinicians.

ARE BEDSIDE SKILLS AND COMPASSION PRACTICAL TO TEACH?

There has been a long-term debate whether compassion can be taught. Some argue that compassion is an innate quality of character.[2] Current evidence suggests that compassion can be developed and sustained over time.[2] At the beginning of training, students demonstrate different levels of inherent compassion. Subsequently, capacity varies from student to student depending on their character at the baseline.[2] Recently, a randomized controlled trial on empathy training suggested that inherent qualities can be developed and sustained.[3]

Eight observational studies focused on educational interventions aimed at improving compassionate care provided by clinicians and students in a clinical setting.[4-12] The researchers used a variety methods (journals, simulations, reflection, etc.) and found that students demonstrate improved self-awareness, clinical communication skills, job satisfaction, caregiving competence, satisfaction with provision, and caregiver and workplace wellness.[4-12] Considering these results, it is safe to suggest that compassion is teachable.

Another group of authors found that common exemplary characteristics can improve humanistic behavior. Some of these were nonverbal communication, overt demonstrations of respect, building a personal connection, and eliciting and addressing patients' affective response to illness.[13] The authors concluded that there are many ways clinical teachers demonstrate humanistic behavior at the bedside.[13] Collectively, these findings suggest that as medical educators we have a role to play in teaching by example: Our humanistic behavior will build the same in students.[14] I am optimistic that the Insight from the PCP section of this book will reveal the art of medicine and be a valuable resource to promote a love of humanity.

CONCLUSION

Humanism and competent care are the primary focus of this book. If you are a PA, NP, or medical student, this will be a helpful and practical workbook during your education. These are real cases, so you know exactly what took place and how the cases were managed. To protect patients' privacy, names and other identifying information have been omitted, and some details about the cases were changed. Additionally, the authors who treated these patients do not have a byline on the case to further protect patient privacy. My goal is to share the practical aspect from each case and provide you an excellent learning opportunity while protecting every patient's privacy. Working through this book prior to clinical clerkships will provide a good foundation. Also, for practicing PCPs or clinicians about to enter practice, this book will be a helpful and practical resource.

When treating a patient, a PCP has an opportunity to provide comprehensive care that is both evidenced based and compassionate. All of us practicing clinicians and/or medical educators and future clinicians should be deliberate in our efforts to provide comprehensive care. It is my sincere hope that *101 Primary Care Case Studies* will contribute to your ability to be a compassionate and competent PCP. Be well.

Sampath ("Sam") Wijesinghe

REFERENCES

1. Sinclair S, Torres MB, Raffin-Bouchal S, et al. Compassion training in healthcare: what are patients' perspectives on training healthcare providers? *BMC Med Educ.* 2016;16:169. doi:10.1186/s12909-016-0695-0
2. American Medical Association. Code of medical ethics. Principle 1. 2001. https://www.ama-assn.org/sites/ama-assn.org/files/corp/media-browser/principles-of-medical-ethics.pdf
3. Sinclair S, Norris JM, McConnell SJ, et al. Compassion: a scoping review of the healthcare literature. *BMC Palliat Care.* 2016;15:6. doi:10.1186/s12904-016-0080-0
4. Riess H, Kelley JM, Bailey RW, et al. Empathy training for resident physicians: a randomized controlled trial of a neuroscience-informed curriculum. *J Gen Intern Med.* 2012;27(10):1280–1286. doi:10.1007/s11606-012-2063-z
5. Adamson E, Dewar B. Compassionate care: student nurses' learning through reflection and the use of story. *Nurse Educ Pract.* 2014;15(3):155–161. doi:10.1016/j.nepr.2014.08.002
6. Betcher DK. Elephant in the room project: improving caring efficacy through effective and compassionate communication with palliative care patients. *Medsurg Nurs.* 2010;19(2):101–105.
7. Blanco MA, Maderer A, Price LL, et al. Efficiency is not enough; you have to prove that you care: role modelling of compassionate care in an innovative resident-as-teacher initiative. *Educ Health (Abingdon).* 2013;26(1):60–65. doi:10.4103/1357-6283.112805
8. Deloney LA, Graham CJ. Wit: using drama to teach first-year medical students about empathy and compassion. *Teach Learn Med.* 2003;15(4):247–251. doi:10.1207/s15328015tlm1504_06
9. Dewar B, Cook F. Developing compassion through a relationship centred appreciative leadership programme. *Nurse Educ Today.* 2014;34(9):1258–1264. doi:10.1016/j.nedt.2013.12.012
10. Fortney L, Luchterhand C, Zakletskaia L, et al. Abbreviated mindfulness intervention for job satisfaction, quality of life, and compassion in primary care clinicians: a pilot study. *Ann Fam Med.* 2013;11(5):412–420. doi:10.1370/afm.1511
11. Kalish R, Dawiskiba M, Sung YC, Blanco M. Raising medical student awareness of compassionate care through reflection of annotated videotapes of clinical encounters. *Educ Health (Abingdon).* 2011;24(3):490.
12. Shih CY, Hu WY, Lee LT, et al. Effect of a compassion-focused training program in palliative care education for medical students. *Am J Hosp Palliat Care.* 2013;30(2):114–120. doi:10.1177/1049909112445463.
13. Weissmann PF, Branch WT, Gracey CF, et al. Role modeling humanistic behavior: learning bedside manner from the experts. *Acad Med J Assoc Am Med Coll.* 2006;81(7):661–667. doi:10.1097/01.ACM.0000232423.81299.fe
14. Institute of Medicine. *Improving Medical Education: Enhancing the Behavioral and Social Science Content of Medical School Curricula.* National Academies Press; 2004.

ACKNOWLEDGMENTS

I want to thank the Springer Publishing Company for the opportunity to publish this book. Particularly, I would like to thank my editor, Suzanne Toppy, for her patience and sound guidance.

A total of 26 physician assistants, 12 nurse practitioners, and 13 physicians have contributed cases for this publication. Also, 25 PAs, 3 NPs, 5 physicians, and 1 psychologist have served as peer reviewers. Thank you for your contributions and reviews.

A special thank you to the following individuals:

- Dr. Dan Fernando and Dr. Thomas Jayawardane for inspiring me to pursue my advanced degree and reinforcing that the United States was the best place to reach my goals
- Mr. D. Ratnayake and Mrs. Celine Ratnayake for standing by me when I really needed them
- Dr. Derrick Gruen for suggesting to me that primary care medicine is the best fit for my personality
- Dr. Sue Fernandes and Dr. Gerald Kayingo for believing in me as a PA educator
- Dr. Virginia Hass for her expertise and editorial support
- Dr. Ade Anast for her editorial support from beginning to end. I wouldn't have completed this book without your help.

HOW TO USE THIS BOOK

- Cases are organized randomly in the table of contents by a patient's chief complaint, which is how a patient realistically presents in clinic.
- You will work through real-life patient cases* and answer a series of questions to determine the workup, diagnosis, and treatment for a patient. Except for question 6, the questions in each case are the same, to help guide you on how to methodically work through a patient's complaint. The questions are as follows:

1. **What is the differential diagnosis?** Pay careful attention to the history of present illness, review of systems, relevant history, and physical exam to determine a list of differential diagnoses. Provide a rationale for each diagnosis on your list. Briefly explain why or why not it is the most likely diagnosis.

2. **What is the most likely diagnosis? Why?** Based on the information available, determine the most likely diagnosis. Some cases are straightforward; others are not. That is the reality in primary care. Keep in mind you are making a most likely diagnosis, not a definitive diagnosis.

3. **Demonstrate your understanding about the pathophysiology in regard to the most likely diagnosis.** While this is not a focus of the book, it is practical to have a basic understanding of a disease.

4. **Should tests/imaging studies be ordered? Which ones? Why? Think about tests/imaging beyond the primary care setting as well.** Determine what diagnostic testing and/or imaging is needed to evaluate the patient. What tests will be performed in the clinic? What tests or images might you want to order but are not typically available in a primary care setting? The online supplement provides details about the tests/imaging ordered by the primary care provider (PCP) and other specialists involved in the case and also provides the results.

5. **What are the next appropriate steps in management?** Think about what your next steps would be for this patient. Are you going to treat and manage the patient? Would you transfer the patient to the ED? Would you refer to a specialist? If you are unclear how to move forward, check the online supplement to determine your progress and then move forward as appropriate.

6. **Review research on the diagnosis. Provide reference(s).** This question will vary from case to case, asking about risk factors, diagnostic criteria, prevalence, treatment options, and other information about the diagnosis under consideration. The use of evidence-based medicine is essential to stay abreast of recent developments, and no one has a greater need for an incredibly broad and deep knowledge base than a PCP. Read and rely on the best available research and refer to evidence whenever it is available. This, coupled with growing clinical expertise, is essential for practicing medicine. We are all lifelong learners.

7. **What are the pertinent ICD-10 and CPT (E/M) codes for this visit? Provide a short rationale.** ICD-10 has approximately 68,000 codes. Medical practitioners are expected to

be specific when choosing these codes. This is an opportunity for future clinicians to learn how to do this. In addition, CPT (E/M) coding can be challenging for new clinicians. If there is an established patient with a medical diagnosis, clinicians may find it challenging to determine whether the visit is coded as level 3 or level 4. This exercise builds this skill. Remember to use the diagnostic codes for the initial visit.

8. **What is the appropriate patient education for this case?** PCPs have a responsibility to educate patients on disease, diagnosis, treatment, and good health habits. This is mandatory and part of every patient visit.

9. **If not managed appropriately, what is/are the medical/legal concern(s) that may arise?** Despite training and experience, there are rare occasions when a negative patient outcome or experience leads to legal action or medical consequence. It is important that young clinicians identify areas of legal exposure and the consequences of incorrect diagnoses and negligence.

10. **Think about interprofessional collaboration for this case. Provide a list of specialties or other disciplines and indicate what contribution these professionals might make to managing the patient.** Medicine is a team sport. PCPs cannot do their jobs alone. It is essential that clinicians value each team member and recognize their contributions. This question will help you become aware of how many individuals actually contribute to a patient's care.

- The cases conclude with a few questions (11–13, but not all three are always included) about your personal bedside manner approach, including communication, handling a distressed patient or parent, and dealing with negative outcomes. These are subjective questions for which answers are not directly provided, but are intended to be thought-provoking and to encourage discussion.
- Pay careful attention to the history of present illness, review of systems, relevant history, and physical exam to determine the best answers to these questions.
- Answers to all the questions are available on Springer Publishing Connect. Instructions for how to access Connect appears on the Connect access card that accompanies this book. Try to answer the questions yourself before reviewing the answers and outcomes online.
- Note that the answers for the bedside manner questions are somewhat subjective. The Outcome and Insight from the PCP sections in the online supplement demonstrate the author's bedside manner and compassion and how the case developed and concluded. The insights from the PCPs provide valuable information about effective communication skills and ways to build trust and underscore the importance of a PCP–patient relationship.
- Keep in mind that medicine is subjective, and clinicians have different approaches to managing patients. They may come up with the same diagnosis at the end; however, their approaches will likely differ.
- For instructors who are using this workbook in a classroom environment, a filterable table of contents is available to you to sort through cases by diagnosis, patient population, gender, and organ system to aid in assignments. Contact your Springer Publishing sales representative for access at springerpub.com/instructors.
- A breakdown of the number of cases by systems appears below:

○	Behavioral Medicine	5	○	Infectious Disease/ Reproductive System	4
○	Cardiovascular System	5	○	Infectious Disease	10
○	Dermatologic System	5	○	Musculoskeletal System	12
○	Endocrine System	7	○	Neurologic System	7
○	Eyes, Ears, Nose, and Throat	8	○	Pulmonary System	8
○	Gastrointestinal System	11	○	Renal System	5
○	Genitourinary System	4	○	Reproductive System	5
○	Hematology/Oncology	5			

*Demographics and patient data have been altered to protect privacy.

ANKLE AND CALF PAIN, ADULT MALE

CHIEF COMPLAINT

"Ankle and calf pain."

HISTORY OF PRESENT ILLNESS

A 51-year-old man presents with a 2-hour-old right ankle and calf injury. He is a firefighter, married, father of teenaged boys, ages 15, 13, and 10 years. He reports he was trying to push his stalled car from out in the street when he heard a pop near his right ankle. He immediately fell to the ground in pain. When he tried to stand up and walk, he was unable to push off the ground with his right ankle and foot. He is unable to walk normally. He noticed immediate swelling at the back of his right heel bone and in the calf muscle. He denies right foot or ankle pain and also has no tingling, numbness, or weakness in the right leg, calf, or foot. He describes the pain as 8/10 when the injury happened, but now the pain has subsided to 2/10. The pain is relieved by rest and elevation of the right ankle and leg. It is made worse by putting weight on the right leg. He denies any prior injury to the right lower extremity, denies recent long-distance travel or sedentary lifestyle, denies any recent or remote steroid use, and denies recent antibiotic use.

REVIEW OF SYSTEMS

The patient's ROS is positive for pain and swelling in the back of his right heel. His review of systems is negative for chest pain, SOB, fatigue, fever, chills, joint pain, numbness or tingling to the right leg/calf, or muscle weakness.

RELEVANT HISTORY

The patient's history is significant for degenerative disc disease of the cervical spine. He drinks three beers per week but denies any smoking or illicit drug use. He is sexually active. He lives with his wife and children and describes his marriage as happy. Both his parents are alive; his father is alive, aged 73, with hypertension. His mother is 70 years old, with bilateral knee osteoarthritis.

ALLERGIES

No known drug allergies; no known food allergies.

MEDICATIONS

Ibuprofen 200 mg 2 tablets every 6 hours PO since the injury occurred.

PHYSICAL EXAMINATION

Vitals: T 37°C (98.6°F), P 68, R 16, BP 132/78, HT 185.4 cm (73 in.), WT 86 kg (191 lbs), BMI 25.2.

General: Appears conversant and uncomfortable.

Psychiatric: Exhibiting anxiousness.

Skin, Hair, and Nails: No obvious lesions, warm, no signs of infection.

Lungs: Clear to auscultation bilaterally.

Heart: RRR, without murmur or gallop.

Musculoskeletal: His right patella appears atraumatic. The patellar tendon is not tender. His knee exhibits full active range of motion 0 to 130 degrees. No knee edema or effusion noted. No crepitus palpated, nor any joint line tenderness elicited medially or laterally. Negative varus, valgus, anterior and posterior drawer testing. Negative Lachman testing. McMurray test is negative.

Edema noted posteriorly mid-calf with obvious bunching of the muscles. There is a palpable defect and tenderness 5 cm proximal to the insertion of the Achilles tendon on the calcaneus.

The right ankle appears atraumatic, no edema or deformity, non-tender to medial and lateral malleoli. The medial ligaments are non-tender to palpation. The lateral ligaments are non-tender to palpation. There is full active dorsiflexion of the right ankle. There is no active plantarflexion of the right ankle. A Thompson test is performed and is positive. An ankle anterior drawer test is negative.

His right foot appears atraumatic, with no edema or deformity. The right tarsals, metatarsals, and phalanges are palpated and are non-tender. The patient can invert and evert the foot without deficit, along with full plantar and dorsiflexion of the toes. Circulation of the dorsalis pedis artery is 2+.

Neurologic: A&O×3. The sensory examination of the right lower extremity reveals intact light touch to all of the right lower extremity, and sharp/dull testing to the plantar and dorsal aspects of the right foot is fully intact.

CLINICAL DISCUSSION QUESTIONS

1. What is the differential diagnosis?

_____

_____

_____

_____

2. What is the most likely diagnosis? Why?

_____

_____

_____

_____

3. Demonstrate your understanding about the pathophysiology in regard to the most likely diagnosis.

_____

_____

_____

_____

4. Should tests/imaging studies be ordered? Which ones? Why? Think about tests/imaging beyond the primary care setting as well.

_____

_____

_____

_____

5. What are the next appropriate steps in management?

_____

_____

_____

_____

6. Review a credible research article on the role of ultrasound in the diagnosis. Demonstrate your understanding of the role of ultrasound versus MRI in the diagnosis. Provide references for your response.

_____

_____

_____

_____

7. What are the pertinent ICD-10 and CPT (E/M) codes for this visit? Provide a short rationale.

_____

_____

_____

_____

8. What is the appropriate patient education for this case?

_____

_____

_____

_____

9. If not managed appropriately, what is/are the medical/legal concern(s) that may arise?

_____

_____

_____

_____

10. Think about interprofessional collaboration for this case. Provide a list of specialties or other disciplines and indicate what contribution these professionals might make to managing the patient.

_____

_____

_____

_____

BEDSIDE MANNER QUESTION

11. How would you communicate your likely diagnosis to the patient?

_____

_____

_____

_____

 ANSWER KEY _available at_
https://connect.springerpub.com/content/book/978-0-8261-8273-9

FATIGUE AND WEAKNESS, ADULT FEMALE

CHIEF COMPLAINT
"Fatigue and weakness."

HISTORY OF PRESENT ILLNESS
A 52-year-old Caucasian woman presents to her PCP with complaints of increasing fatigue and weakness over the past 3 to 4 months. She is an avid runner and finds it difficult to keep her usual distance or pace. She tried adding a multivitamin to her daily regimen and has been tracking her sleep on an exercise-tracking watch for the past month without significant findings. She does report having some irregularity with her menses over this past year, but her routine gynecologic exam showed no significant concerns and she denies excessive or heavy bleeding. Her gynecologist reportedly told her she is likely in perimenopause after confirming she is not pregnant with an in-office urine hCG, and she has a follow-up appointment scheduled in about 6 weeks. The patient denies any anxiety or depression and reports good social activity. Her diet is vegetarian and reported as well balanced.

REVIEW OF SYSTEMS
The patient's ROS is positive for asthenia without anorexia or weight loss and positive for angular cheilosis and increased soreness of tongue and mouth at times, and she does note some mild hair loss and brittle nails. Her ROS is also positive for some dyspnea on exertion and exercise intolerance, and she has some constipation. She denies chest pain or palpitations. The ROS is also negative for abdominal pain, nausea, vomiting, or diarrhea. She denies blood in stools, hematuria, or dysuria. The patient also denies dizziness, blurred vision, headache, anxiety, and depression. She denies fever, chills, and night sweats and has had no significant change in weight or unusual bruising reported.

RELEVANT HISTORY
The patient's history is unremarkable. Her menses are irregular, less frequent for the past 9 months, with her last menstrual period about 8 weeks ago without excessive or heavy bleeding. Her surgical history is significant for one cesarean section at age 28 and appendectomy at age 35.

The patient is married and lives at home with her spouse and youngest child. She is employed as an accountant full-time with a graduate school education. She denies smoking or illicit drug use. She drinks socially, reporting about four to five glasses of wine per week. Her family history includes her mother, aged 76 with hypertension, and father, aged 77 with hyperlipidemia, hypertension, and gout.

ALLERGIES
Fluoroquinolones-rash; no known food allergies.

MEDICATIONS
- Women's over-50 multivitamin.
- Ooccasional ibuprofen 400 mg PRN for pain.

PHYSICAL EXAMINATION

Vitals: T 36°C (96.8°F), P 62, R 14, BP 112/62; HT 170 cm (67 in.), WT 57 kg (126 lbs), BMI 19.4.

General: A&O×3, well groomed.

Psychiatric: Normal affect, pleasant and cooperative.

Skin, Hair, and Nails: Skin dry but without rash or lesions, normal hair distribution, brittle nails.

Eye: Mild pallor of conjunctiva.

ENT/Mouth: Evidence of healing angular cheilosis bilaterally with some smoothness and redness of tongue. Mucous membranes with some mild pallor.

Neck: Supple without thyromegaly. Head and neck lymph nodes within normal limits.

Lungs: Clear to auscultation with normal respiratory effort.

Heart: S1S2, RRR; no murmur noted.

Abdomen: Soft, nontender, no distention. No organomegaly. Positive and normal bowel sounds in all quadrants.

Genital/Rectal: No external hemorrhoids, negative for occult blood. Genital exam deferred.

Neurologic: CN II–XII grossly intact with normal patellar deep tendon reflexes.

CLINICAL DISCUSSION QUESTIONS

1. What is the differential diagnosis?

_____

_____

_____

_____

2. What is the most likely diagnosis? Why?

_____

_____

_____

_____

3. Demonstrate your understanding about the pathophysiology in regard to the most likely diagnosis.

_____

_____

_____

_____

4. Should tests/imaging studies be ordered? Which ones? Why? Think about tests/imaging beyond the primary care setting as well.

_____

_____

_____

_____

5. What are the next appropriate steps in management?

_____

_____

_____

_____

6. What are the causes, risk factors, and treatment options for this diagnosis? Provide references for your response.

_____

_____

_____

_____

7. What are the pertinent ICD-10 and CPT (E/M) codes for this visit? Provide a short rationale.

_____

_____

_____

_____

8. What is the appropriate patient education for this case?

_____

_____

_____

_____

9. If not managed appropriately, what is/are the medical/legal concern(s) that may arise?

_____

_____

_____

_____

10. Think about interprofessional collaboration for this case. Provide a list of specialties or other disciplines and indicate what contribution these professionals might make to managing the patient.

_____

_____

_____

_____

BEDSIDE MANNER QUESTIONS

11. How would you communicate your likely diagnosis to the patient?

_____

_____

_____

_____

12. If the patient shows distress at what you communicate, how would you provide support?

_____

_____

_____

_____

ANSWER KEY *available at*
https://connect.springerpub.com/content/book/978-0-8261-8273-9

ABDOMINAL PAIN, ADOLESCENT MALE

CHIEF COMPLAINT

"Abdominal pain."

HISTORY OF PRESENT ILLNESS

A 17-year-old boy presents to his PCP with abdominal pain, nausea, vomiting, poor appetite, headache, and diarrhea. He has been sick since last night. He describes his abdominal pain as "really bad" and states his pain level as 5/10. He states, "I don't know how to describe the pain, but I know it's really bad." He points to the entire abdomen as the location of the pain. When asked where the pain started, he states, "The entire stomach." He vomited once this afternoon and is now nauseous. He states he had loose stool this morning. He indicates that "most likely it was diarrhea this morning; but I am not 100% sure." He further states, "I do have loose stools a lot." He denies fever, chills, cough, runny nose, sore throat, abdominal bloating, acid reflux, neck stiffness, urinary urgency, dysuria, hematochezia, back pain, wheezing, SOB, recent travel, new medication, or known sick contacts, including home and school. He does not recall eating or drinking anything out of ordinary. He has been eating and drinking almost the same food and drinks as the entire family. He has been taking acetaminophen 500 mg every 6 hours to manage his pain, and it has helped his pain slightly. He is here today with his older sister, who drove him to the appointment.

REVIEW OF SYSTEMS

His ROS is positive for abdominal pain, nausea, and vomiting. He reports headache and lack of appetite. The ROS is questionable for diarrhea. The ROS is negative for fever, chills, constipation, cough, runny nose, sore throat, abdominal bloating, acid reflux, neck stiffness, urinary urgency, dysuria, hematochezia, back pain, wheezing, SOB, or chest pain.

RELEVANT HISTORY

The patient's medical history is significant for acne (onset age 14), obesity, hepatic steatosis, and mild intermittent asthma (onset age 8). He has no surgical history. His social history includes playing football and traveling with his family. He has two sisters and two brothers. He lives with his father and does not have much interaction with his mom. He has been sexually active since age 16 with one female partner. He uses condoms. His family history includes diabetes (paternal grandparents), hypertension (father), and prostate cancer (paternal grandfather). He does not know his maternal family history.

ALLERGIES

No known drug allergies; no known food allergies.

MEDICATIONS

- Benzoyl peroxide 4% topical QD.
- Albuterol inhaler 2 puffs every 4–6 hours PRN.

Physical Examination

Vitals: T 37.5°C (99.5°F), P 93, R 19, BP 130/87, WT 95.25 kg (210 lbs), HT 177.8 cm (70 in.), BMI 30.1.

General: Mild to moderate distress, obese.

Psychiatric: Cooperative, appropriate mood and affect.

Eyes: Conjunctiva and sclera clear.

ENT/Mouth: Within normal limit.

Neck: Supple, FROM.

Lungs: Clear to auscultation bilaterally.

Heart: Normal rate, regular rhythm, no heart murmur.

Abdomen: Tender abdomen throughout; greatest tenderness in right lower quadrant—guarding even with mild palpation; McBurney point tenderness noted; psoas sign +; Rovsing sign questionable.

Neurologic: A&O×3.

Clinical Discussion Questions

1. What is the differential diagnosis?

_____

_____

_____

_____

2. What is the most likely diagnosis? Why?

_____

_____

_____

_____

3. Demonstrate your understanding about the pathophysiology in regard to the most likely diagnosis.

_____

_____

_____

_____

4. Should tests/imaging studies be ordered? Which ones? Why? Think about tests/imaging beyond the primary care setting as well.

_____

_____

_____

_____

5. What are the next appropriate steps in management?

_____

_____

_____

_____

6. Demonstrate your understanding of the prevalence, diagnostic criteria, and treatment options. Include a list of your reference(s).

_____

_____

_____

_____

7. What are the pertinent ICD-10 and CPT (E/M) codes for this visit? Provide a short rationale.

_____

_____

_____

_____

8. What is the appropriate patient education for this case?

_____

_____

_____

_____

9. If not managed appropriately, what is/are the medical/legal concern(s) that may arise?

_____

_____

_____

_____

10. Think about interprofessional collaboration for this case. Provide a list of specialties or other disciplines and indicate what contribution these professionals might make to managing the patient.

_____

_____

_____

_____

Bedside Manner Questions

11. What would your communication style/approach be with this patient and his sister?

_____

_____

_____

_____

12. If a patient and his sister are distressed by the diagnosis, what might offer support?

_____

_____

_____

_____

Answer Key *available at*
https://connect.springerpub.com/content/book/978-0-8261-8273-9

LEFT HIP PAIN, ADULT FEMALE

CHIEF COMPLAINT
"Left hip pain."

HISTORY OF PRESENT ILLNESS

A 55-year-old woman presents with an ongoing complaint of left hip pain. She had been doing physical therapy as ordered and is back to the office to learn her x-ray results.

Her initial injury was approximately 2 months prior when she had come in with concern about an inguinal/groin strain. She was working full-time as a medical assistant for a local home health agency. On the day of the injury, she heard a pop in her left hip while transferring an older adult patient. Her groin felt tight, "like a vise around my pelvis," but she was able to continue working for another 6 weeks. She came to the clinic initially with a request for physical therapy. She was also started on ibuprofen 600 mg by mouth, three times a day.

She returned to the clinic after 3 weeks and saw a different provider. Her physical therapist shifted emphasis from her groin to her left hip, but this did not help, and she reported that "the pain was worse" following exercise. The provider prescribed low-dose narcotics and a muscle relaxant. A left hip x-ray was ordered, as well as a pelvic ultrasound and x-ray of the lumbar spine.

The patient then sent the PCP an electronic message through her electronic health record requesting short-term disability because she did not feel safe lifting or transferring bed-bound patients.

Prior to her injury, she had been going to the gym three times per week to lift weights but denies any activity that may have hurt her hip in the past. She was a long-distance runner 5 years ago but stopped because of time constraints. She is single, has two adult children, and is normally healthy.

Her last laboratory tests, performed 3 months before injury, were in the normal range.

REVIEW OF SYSTEMS

The patient's ROS is positive for left hip pain with active range of motion and constipation when using narcotics. The ROS is negative for limping, numbness, or tingling in the left foot, and she has no back pain.

RELEVANT HISTORY

Her medical history is significant for childhood asthma (unknown treatment), trigger finger and arthritis in left thumb (age 48), heartburn (age 50), varicose veins in the bilateral lower extremities (age 52), and pain in both feet (age 54). Her surgical history includes a tubal ligation and a right thumb trigger release. The patient was a previous smoker (23 pack years) but quit 12 years ago. She rarely drinks alcohol and uses no recreational drugs. She has not been sexually active for "a couple of years." She lives alone, exercises regularly, and has two grown children. Her family history is positive for mesothelioma (deceased father), obesity, type 2 diabetes (deceased mother), and lung cancer (deceased grandfather).

ALLERGIES

Erythromycin—stomach upset.

MEDICATIONS

Ibuprofen 600 mg PO TID PRN pain.

Physical Examination

Vitals: T 36.4°C (97.6°F), P 78, R 16, BP 116/72, HT 172.5 cm (68 in.), WT 72.6 kg (160 lbs), SpO_2 99% (room air), BMI 24.14.

General: Well-appearing female, mild discomfort with movement in and out of sitting position. Appears stated age.

Psychiatric: Mildly anxious.

Skin, Hair, and Nails: Skin normal in appearance, no rashes or lesions. Normal hair distribution. Nail beds pink with no cyanosis/clubbing.

Head: Normal shape and appearance.

Eyes: Conjunctivae are clear without exudates or hemorrhage. Sclera is non-icteric. Bilateral. Extraocular muscle intact; pupils equal, round, and reactive to light and accommodation. Eyelids are normal in appearance without swelling or lesions.

ENT/Mouth: The external ears are non-tender and without swelling; hearing grossly intact. Nose has no obstruction or discharge. Oropharynx has no inflammation, swelling, exudate or lesion. Mouth with no lesions; dentition good.

Neck: Supple with no adenopathy.

Lungs: Lung sounds clear in all lobes.

Heart: Rate and rhythm are normal.

Abdomen: Soft, non-tender, no masses or guarding.

Musculoskeletal: Leg length equal; sacroiliac stress tests positive for three of five tests: distraction, no pain; thigh thrust, no pain; FABER, positive for pain. Compression, positive for pain. Gaenslen's maneuver, positive for pain. Gait without limp.

Neurologic: Alert/oriented to person/place/time, color/sensation/movement within normal limits on bilateral legs and feet.

Clinical Discussion Questions

1. What is the differential diagnosis?

_____

_____

_____

_____

2. What is the most likely diagnosis? Why?

_____

_____

_____

_____

3. Demonstrate your understanding about the pathophysiology in regard to the most likely diagnosis.

_____

_____

_____

_____

4. Should tests/imaging studies be ordered? Which ones? Why? Think about tests/imaging beyond the primary care setting as well.

_____

_____

_____

_____

5. What are the next appropriate steps in management?

_____

_____

_____

_____

6. What are the risk factors, causes, and most common site for this diagnosis? Provide references for your response.

_____

_____

_____

_____

7. What are the pertinent ICD-10 and CPT (E/M) codes for this visit? Provide a short rationale.

_____

_____

_____

_____

8. What is the appropriate patient education for this case?

_____

_____

_____

_____

9. If not managed appropriately, what is/are the medical/legal concern(s) that may arise?

_____

_____

_____

_____

10. Think about interprofessional collaboration for this case. Provide a list of specialties or other disciplines and indicate what contribution these professionals might make to managing the patient.

_____

_____

_____

_____

BEDSIDE MANNER QUESTIONS

11. How would you communicate your likely diagnosis to the patient?

_____

_____

_____

_____

12. If the patient shows distress at what you communicate, how would you provide support?

_____

_____

_____

_____

13. If diagnostic evidence points to a more complicated case that could potentially result in a negative outcome, how would you communicate this possibility?

_____

_____

_____

_____

ANSWER KEY _available at_
https://connect.springerpub.com/content/book/978-0-8261-8273-9

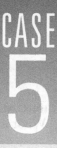

VAGINAL BLEEDING, ADULT FEMALE

CHIEF COMPLAINT
"Vaginal bleeding."

HISTORY OF PRESENT ILLNESS
A 28-year-old woman presents to her PCP with a 3-day history of dizziness, fatigue, and head-ache. She is mother of two girls, ages 5 and 2. She and her husband want another child, hopefully a boy, and have planned accordingly. She missed her last period and suspects she is pregnant; a home pregnancy test last week was positive. Until 3 days ago, she felt fine, other than some fatigue and mild nausea. Over the last 2 days, she began experiencing abdominal cramping and irregular vaginal bleeding. She points to both lower and upper quadrants as the main location of the pain. She describes her abdominal pain as 7 of 10. She has not used over-the-counter pain medication because she wants to avoid medication if pregnant. Additionally, she states, "When changing posi-tions, I get lightheaded." When the PCP asks about her bleeding, she states she has had similar bleeding during her other pregnancies. "All my pregnancies are like that, it's normal."

REVIEW OF SYSTEMS
A ROS is positive for fatigue, nausea, abdominal pain, and vaginal bleeding. The patient reports headache and dizziness. The ROS is negative for fever, chills, vomiting, diarrhea, constipation, shortness of breath, or chest pain.

RELEVANT HISTORY
The patient's medical history is significant for cholecystectomy (age 27) and chlamydia infection (age 17). Her social history includes drinking one glass of wine per weekend since age 18. She had a few male sex partners prior to her marriage. She lives with her husband and children and describes her marriage as happy. Both children were full-term babies and the pregnancies were normal. Her family history is unknown as she was adopted.

ALLERGIES
No known drug allergies; no known food allergies.

MEDICATIONS
None.

PHYSICAL EXAMINATION
Vitals: T 37°C (98.6°F), P 70, R 19, BP 130/80, WT 78.7 kg (173.5 lbs), HT 167.6 cm (66 in.), BMI 28.

General: Appears anxious and fatigued, mild acute distress.

Skin, Hair, and Nails: No rash, skin warm and dry. No abnormal findings with hair or nails.

Lungs: Clear to auscultation bilaterally, good air movement throughout.

Heart: RRR, without murmur or gallop.

> *Abdomen:* Abdomen was soft, non-distended, and moderately tender; generalized.
>
> *Neurologic:* A&O×3, cranial nerves II to XII grossly intact.

CLINICAL DISCUSSION QUESTIONS

1. What is the differential diagnosis?

_____

_____

_____

2. What is the most likely diagnosis? Why?

_____

_____

_____

3. Demonstrate your understanding about the pathophysiology in regard to the most likely diagnosis.

_____

_____

_____

4. Should tests/imaging studies be ordered? Which ones? Why? Think about tests/imaging beyond the primary care setting as well.

_____

_____

_____

5. What are the next appropriate steps in management?

_____

_____

_____

6. Demonstrate your understanding about the most common location of the diagnosis, risk factors, and treatment options. Provide reference for your responses.

_____

_____

_____

7. What are the pertinent ICD-10 and CPT (E/M) codes for this visit? Provide a short rationale.

_____

_____

_____

_____

8. What is the appropriate patient education for this case?

_____

_____

_____

_____

9. If not managed appropriately, what is/are the medical/legal concern(s) that may arise?

_____

_____

_____

_____

10. Think about interprofessional collaboration for this case. Provide a list of specialties or other disciplines and indicate what contribution these professionals might make to managing the patient.

_____

_____

_____

_____

BEDSIDE MANNER QUESTIONS

11. What would your communication style/approach be with this patient?

_____

_____

_____

_____

12. If a patient is distressed by the diagnosis, what might offer support?

_____

_____

_____

_____

ANSWER KEY _available at_
https://connect.springerpub.com/content/book/978-0-8261-8273-9

NUMBNESS IN HANDS AND LEGS, GERIATRIC MALE

CHIEF COMPLAINT

"Numbness in hands and legs."

HISTORY OF PRESENT ILLNESS

A 65-year-old man presents to his PCP with an initial complaint of insidious onset of hand and leg numbness and weakness. He describes tingling and weakness over the last 3 days. He has numbness in a glove-like pattern to both hands and distal forearms, as well as numbness and weakness to his lower extremities. He admits to dropping items now and cannot shake off the tingling and sense of imbalance because of the numbness in his feet. The patient admits to having difficulty getting out of his recliner. He describes progressive and worsening numbness and weakness just over the last day. He also admits to precedent pain to extremities prior to onset of numbness. He has pain in his upper and lower limbs that he describes as a dull, non-radiating ache with severity 5 to 6 of 10, at its worst. The patient states the discomfort has interfered with his sleep, contributing to his fatigue. He has a history of motor vehicle accident, 15 years ago, when his car was rear-ended, and he sustained a lower back and whiplash injury. He states after a year of physical therapy, his painful condition resolved and he was able to resume work. The patient states, "My neck and back pain had been fine for years until 5 days ago." He has no prior surgeries to back or upper extremities. He admits to recent illness, about 3 weeks ago, which he describes as bad "food poisoning" and experienced diarrhea for 5 days with malaise, fatigue, and weight loss of 10 lbs. He was seen by urgent care, closer to home, and was reassured that he had an occurrence of viral gastroenteritis. Since then, he has been fatigued with loss of appetite and been unable to regain his 10-lb weight loss. He states, "It hit me hard and sapped the energy out of me." The patient is here today with his wife.

REVIEW OF SYSTEMS

A ROS is positive for decreased appetite, fatigue, nausea, insomnia, occasional dizziness, and some mild blurring of vision and imbalance problems related to numbness, weakness, and tingling of feet. He denies fever, chills, nausea, vomiting, worsening of chronic headaches, tinnitus, diplopia, dysphagia, SOB, dyspnea on exertion, orthopnea, chest pain, palpitations, paroxysmal nocturnal dyspnea, abdominal pain, current diarrhea, or constipation. The patient has good bowel and bladder control.

RELEVANT HISTORY

The patient's medical history is significant for well-controlled hypertension and hyperlipidemia. He had musculoskeletal neck and back pain for a year after a car accident and was treated conservatively to resolution.

The patient is married with two children and works for the postal service. Active prior to the recent illness, he enjoyed hiking and biking at least once a week with his wife. He does not smoke and has one glass of wine with dinner each evening. He has no history of recreational drug use. He had the usual childhood illnesses. His family history is noncontributory except for a mother with lupus.

ALLERGIES

No known drug allergies; no known food allergies.

MEDICATIONS

- Lisinopril 20 mg PO QD.
- Atorvastatin 20 mg PO QHS.
- Daily multivitamin.

PHYSICAL EXAMINATION

Vitals: T 37°C (98.6°F), P 98, R 14, BP 140/90, WT 82.5 kg (182 lbs), HT 175 cm (69 in.), BMI 27.

General: The patient is in no apparent distress and is ambulatory without an assistive device. He has a slightly ataxic gait and holds onto hallway rails.

Psychiatric: Alert, oriented, and conversant individual. Good historian. Good judgment and insight.

Skin, Hair, and Nails: No lesions, rashes. Hair and nails unremarkable. Hair present to lower extremities and dorsum feet, with even distribution bilaterally.

Head: Normocephalic. Atraumatic.

Eyes: PERRLA. EOMI.

ENT/Mouth: Oral mucosa with good dentition. Gross hearing intact. Bilateral tympanic membrane intact and not inflamed.

Neck: FROM. Trachea midline. No adenopathy.

Chest: Symmetrical. No axillary adenopathy.

Lungs: Bilateral clear lung fields with good air movement.

Heart: RRR, without murmur or gallop.

Abdomen: Abdomen soft, non-tender, bowel sounds intact in all quadrants. No discernible organomegaly.

Genital/Rectal: No anal lesions. Good sphincter tone. Normal male genitalia.

Musculoskeletal: Mild bilateral paraspinous tenderness with deep palpation to base of neck extending to the mid interscapular areas and laterally to posterior shoulders. No nuchal rigidity. No scapular winging. Full active range of motion to neck and shoulder with end range discomfort. Bilateral hands warm and dry. Allen's test negative. Grasp equal but weak symmetrically. No intrinsic muscle wasting noted. Tinel's noted with pain elicited to forearm. Phalen's negative. Hypoesthesia both dorsal and volar aspects of hand extending to wrist in glove-like pattern.

  Lower lumbosacral spine without tenderness. Straight leg raises negative bilaterally. Lhermitte's negative. Lower extremities with active FROM. Motor 4/5 to knees and 4/5 ankles. Hypoesthesia to bilateral feet and ankles extending to distal calf in glove-like pattern with poor discrimination testing to sharp and dull.

Neurologic: Cranial nerves II to XII grossly intact. No facial paresis noted. Deep tendon reflexes: triceps: 1+; brachioradialis/biceps: absent; radial: absent; patellar: 1+; ankle: absent with reinforcement.

Vascular: Peripheral pulses (dorsalis pedis, posterior tibial, radial and ulnar) all 2+ bilaterally. Normal hair growth in lower and upper extremities with quick capillary refill bilateral toes and fingers.

CLINICAL DISCUSSION QUESTIONS

1. What is the differential diagnosis?

_____

_____

_____

_____

2. What is the most likely diagnosis? Why?

_____

_____

_____

_____

3. Demonstrate your understanding about the pathophysiology in regard to the most likely diagnosis.

_____

_____

_____

_____

4. Should tests/imaging studies be ordered? Which ones? Why? Think about tests/imaging beyond the primary care setting as well.

_____

_____

_____

_____

5. What are the next appropriate steps in management?

_____

_____

_____

_____

6. What are the triggers, associated microorganisms, critical predictors, and complications of the disease? Provide references for your response.

_____

_____

_____

_____

7. What are the pertinent ICD-10 and CPT (E/M) codes for this visit? Provide a short rationale.

_____

_____

_____

_____

8. What are the appropriate patient education topics for this case?

_____

_____

_____

_____

9. If not managed appropriately, what is/are the medical/legal concern(s) that may arise?

_____

_____

_____

_____

10. Think about interprofessional collaboration for this case. Provide a list of specialties or other disciplines and indicate what contribution these professionals might make to managing the patient.

_____

_____

_____

_____

BEDSIDE MANNER QUESTIONS

11. What would your communication style/approach be with this patient and his wife?

_____

_____

_____

_____

12. If a patient and his wife are distressed by the diagnosis, what might offer support?

_____

_____

_____

_____

ANSWER KEY _available at_
https://connect.springerpub.com/content/book/978-0-8261-8273-9

PAINFUL RASH, GERIATRIC MALE

CHIEF COMPLAINT

"Painful rash."

HISTORY OF PRESENT ILLNESS

A 68-year-old man presents to his PCP with a 1-week history of thoracic pain. He describes the pain as slow onset of symptoms on the right side of his thoracic spine radiating to his anterior trunk. The pain has progressively worsened, and he describes it as sharp and burning. He states the discomfort started a week ago as an ache after returning from work. He suspected a strained muscle and treated with warm packs and over-the-counter ibuprofen. In the subsequent days, his pain became worse, and he was concerned he had irreversibly injured his back. He denies any associated paresthesia or recent weight loss.

About 2 days ago, he noticed a mildly pruritic rash to his abdomen, and he was not sure if this was related to his pain. He states, "It even hurts to breathe now," noting that positional changes make the pain worse. He states it is very tender to lay on his right side.

He is a fieldworker; he drives heavy equipment and supervises other workers. He is concerned he injured his back getting in or out of equipment, which occurs frequently during a normal workday.

REVIEW OF SYSTEMS

A ROS is positive for difficulty sleeping related to right upper abdominal pain, fatigue, mild dyspepsia, decreased appetite, and mild dyspnea on exertion related to pain. The ROS is negative for fever, chills, cough, vomiting, sick contacts, melena, hematochezia, liver disease, HIV, headache, dizziness, blurred vision, recent travel requiring prolonged sitting, paroxysmal nocturnal dyspnea, lower extremity, palpitations, paresthesia, or muscle weakness.

RELEVANT HISTORY

The patient's medical history is significant for well-controlled type 2 diabetes, hypertension, hyperlipidemia, and obesity. His surgical history is significant for cholecystectomy (age 48), colonoscopy, and upper endoscopy (age 65) revealing mild gastritis. He admits to usual childhood illnesses. Social history is significant for one to two beers after work daily. The patient quit smoking cigarettes at age 48 and denies recreational drug use. He is heterosexual with no history of sexually transmitted infections and enjoys a monogamous relationship with his wife. He has three grown children, nine grandchildren, and one great grandson. He resides in a single-story home with his wife. He is the primary wage earner. He states a granddaughter is reliant on him for college funding. His family history is unknown.

ALLERGIES

No known drug allergies; no known food allergies.

MEDICATIONS

- Metformin 1,000 mg PO BID.
- Glargine insulin 15 units SQ QD.
- Atorvastatin 20 mg QD.
- Lisinopril 20 mg PO QD.
- Aspirin 81 mg PO QD.
- Fish oil (omega 3) 1,000 mg PO QD.

PHYSICAL EXAMINATION

Vitals: T 37°C (98.6°F), P 88, R 14, BP 138/82, WT 85 kg (188 lbs), HT 170 cm (67 in.), BMI 29.

General: Spanish-speaking male. Grimacing and appears in pain with guarded movements.

Psychiatric: Good historian with linear thought processes.

Skin, Hair, and Nails: Right sub-xiphoid area with 1- to 2cm papular vesicular rash on background of hyperemia in clusters, extending laterally to midclavicular line in dermatomal pattern. Few dispersed vesicles noted. No lymphadenopathy to axilla. No other lesions or rashes noted. Hair and nails unremarkable. Hair present to lower extremities and dorsum feet, with even distribution bilaterally.

Head: Normocephalic, atraumatic.

Eyes: PERRLA, EOMI.

ENT/Mouth: Dentition in good repair. Gross hearing intact. Bilateral TMs patent.

Neck: FROM, trachea midline, no adenopathy.

Chest: Symmetrical, no axillary adenopathy.

Lungs: Clear to auscultation bilaterally. Good air movement discernible.

Heart: RRR, without murmur/gallop.

Back: No spinous tenderness. Right back tender to touch at approximately T7; inferior angle of scapula level. FROM neck with flexion, extension, lateral and rotational movements. FROM left and right shoulder without scapular winging.

Abdomen: Protuberant. Moderate tenderness right upper quadrant and epigastric area to light touch. No peritoneal signs. No ascites. Murphy sign negative. Negative rebound.

Neurologic: Cranial nerves II to XII intact. Hyperesthesia right T7 to T8 dermatomes; otherwise normal gross motor sensation in upper and lower extremities.

CLINICAL DISCUSSION QUESTIONS

1. What is the differential diagnosis?

_____

_____

_____

_____

2. What is the most likely diagnosis? Why?

_____

_____

_____

_____

3. Demonstrate your understanding about the pathophysiology in regard to the most likely diagnosis.

_____

_____

_____

_____

4. Should tests/imaging studies be ordered? Which ones? Why? Think about tests/imaging beyond the primary care setting as well.

_____

_____

_____

_____

5. What are the next appropriate steps in management?

_____

_____

_____

_____

6. Review reliable articles and investigate the prevalence, treatment options, associated symptom(s), and recurrence of the diagnosis. Include the name of the references.

_____

_____

_____

_____

7. What are the pertinent ICD-10 and CPT (E/M) codes for this visit? Provide a short rationale.

_____

_____

_____

_____

8. What are the appropriate patient education topics for this case?

_____

_____

_____

_____

9. If not managed appropriately, what is/are the medical/legal concern(s) that may arise?

_____

_____

_____

_____

10. Think about interprofessional collaboration for this case. Provide a list of specialties or other disciplines and indicate what contribution these professionals might make to managing the patient.

_____

_____

_____

_____

BEDSIDE MANNER QUESTION

11. What would your communication style/approach be with this patient?

_____

_____

_____

_____

ANSWER KEY *available at*
https://connect.springerpub.com/content/book/978-0-8261-8273-9

FEVER AND BODY ACHES, ADULT MALE

CHIEF COMPLAINT

"Fever and body aches."

HISTORY OF PRESENT ILLNESS

A 27-year-old man presents to his PCP with a history of fever, chills, sore throat, body aches, and headache. He states, "I have been having fevers, chills, fatigue, sore throat, body aches, and headache for the last 4 days. I thought I would be better by now, but I think I am getting worse. I just returned from a vacation in Papua New Guinea. I think I have the seasonal flu or malaria. I did not have a chance to get this year's flu shot or malaria prevention medicine prior to my trip. I need your help please." The patient is a music teacher who loves traveling with a group every winter. About 4 weeks ago, he went on a vacation to tropical New Guinea. He admits to having unprotected sex with a woman in the travel group and unprotected sex with a local man. He is concerned his symptoms are not improving. He has been resting and drinking plenty of fluids. In addition, he has been taking ibuprofen 400 mg every 6 hours as needed for his fever. Ibuprofen has reduced his fever slightly and helped him with his body aches, sore throat, and headache. As the patient states, his fever has been consistent and the only way he can manage it is by taking ibuprofen. He states, "I have some family members with flu-like symptoms and met them for a short time last week during a family event." He denies any other symptoms.

REVIEW OF SYSTEMS

The patient is positive for fevers, chills, sore throat, and body aches. He reports fatigue and headache. The ROS is negative for diarrhea, constipation, nausea, vomiting, rash, runny nose, cough, urinary urgency, dysuria, back pain, abdominal pain, penile discharge, night sweat, diaphoresis, loss of appetite, SOB, or chest pain.

RELEVANT HISTORY

The patient's medical history is significant for an appendectomy (age 15) and gonorrhea (age 23). He has no chronic medical problems. Currently, he is not taking any medication other than ibuprofen. His social history includes drinking eight beers over the weekend. He has had three female sex partners during the last year. His family history includes a father with benign prostatic hyperplasia, hypertension, and type 2 diabetes and mother with type 2 diabetes and breast cancer. His siblings (two sisters and one brother) are younger, and their medical histories are unremarkable.

ALLERGIES

No known drug allergies; no known food allergies.

MEDICATIONS

Ibuprofen 400 mg every 6 hours PRN.

PHYSICAL EXAMINATION

Vitals: T 39.4°C (102.9°F), P 84, R 18, BP 140/89, WT 71.7 kg (158 lbs), HT 172.7 cm (68 in.), BMI 24.

General: Febrile; appears anxious and fatigue; NAD.

Psychiatric: Cooperative; appropriate mood and affect.

Skin, Hair, and Nails: No skin rash or lesions. No abnormal findings with hair and nail exam.

Eyes: Conjunctiva and sclera clear.

ENT/Mouth: In normal limits, except for mild rhinorrhea.

Neck: Bilateral anterior cervical lymphadenopathy; no posterior cervical lymph nodes.

Lungs: Clear with good air movement.

Heart: RRR; no murmur or gallop.

Abdomen: Soft, non-tender, not distended; no organomegaly.

Neurologic: A&O×3.

CLINICAL DISCUSSION QUESTIONS

1. What is the differential diagnosis?

_____

_____

_____

2. What is the most likely diagnosis? Why?

_____

_____

_____

3. Demonstrate your understanding of the pathophysiology in regard to the most likely diagnosis.

_____

_____

_____

4. Should tests/imaging studies be ordered? Which ones? Why? Think about tests/imaging beyond the primary care setting as well.

_____

_____

_____

5. What are the next appropriate steps in management?

_____

_____

_____

_____

6. Review recent and credible research article/s on this diagnosis. Demonstrate your understanding about the transmission, screening tests, and treatment initiation. Provide references for your response(s).

_____

_____

_____

_____

7. What are the pertinent ICD-10 and CPT (E/M) codes for this visit? Provide a short rationale.

_____

_____

_____

_____

8. What is the appropriate patient education for this case?

_____

_____

_____

_____

9. If not managed appropriately, what is/are the medical/legal concern(s) that may arise?

_____

_____

_____

_____

10. Think about interprofessional collaboration for this case. Provide a list of specialties or other disciplines and indicate what contribution these professionals might make to managing the patient.

_____

_____

_____

_____

BEDSIDE MANNER QUESTIONS
11. What would your communication style/approach be with this patient?

_____

_____

_____

_____

12. If a patient is distressed by the diagnosis, what might offer support?

_____

_____

_____

_____

Answer Key _available at_
https://connect.springerpub.com/content/book/978-0-8261-8273-9

FEVER AND RASH, PEDIATRIC MALE

CHIEF COMPLAINT

"Fever and rash."

HISTORY OF PRESENT ILLNESS

An 8-year-old boy accompanied by his mother presents to his PCP with a 4-day history of fever and rash. His mother states the illness began with a runny nose, cough, and pinkeye. The rash started yesterday on his head and spread to his trunk and lower extremities. The patient denies emesis, diarrhea, headache, and photophobia. He is eating and drinking and is intermittently playful. No discharge noted from the eyes. No sore throat or lesions noted by his mother on his lips or in his mouth. He does not have a rash on the palms or soles of feet. His mother states they returned from a family vacation to Europe about 10 days ago. The patient is homeschooled. No other family members or friends have similar symptoms.

REVIEW OF SYSTEMS

A ROS is positive for fatigue. It is negative for nausea, abdominal pain, blood in stool, or changes in urination. No chills or myalgias noted. No chest pain or SOB noted.

RELEVANT HISTORY

His mother was G1P1 and describes a normal pregnancy, labor, and delivery. The child has no surgical history or chronic medical conditions. He had a febrile seizure when he was 9 months old. He was seen in an ED for the seizure, and a subsequent workup was negative. He has had no further seizures. He received vaccines from birth to 6 months, but after the seizure, the mother refused vaccines, fearing they will trigger another seizure. The child lives with his parents and has no siblings. There is no family history of seizure disorders.

ALLERGIES

No known drug allergies; no known food allergies.

MEDICATIONS

None.

PHYSICAL EXAMINATION

Vitals: T 39.5°C (103.2°F), P 105, R 16, BP 98/59, HT 127 cm (50 in.), WT 25.4 kg (56 lbs), BMI 15.7.

General: Well appearing, appropriately responsive, in no acute distress.

Skin, Hair, and Nails: Erythematous, blanching macular-papular rash from hairline to toes. Coalesces on trunk. No petechiae. No involvement of palms or soles.

Eyes: Conjunctiva red bilaterally. No tearing or purulent discharge noted.

ENT/Mouth: Nose with erythematous turbinates and clear-yellow discharge. Post-nasal drip noted. No posterior oropharynx erythema or exudate. Small white spots on erythematous base noted on buccal mucosa. TMs pearly gray and mobile bilaterally.

Neck: Mild anterior cervical lymphadenopathy noted. No thyromegaly or tenderness to palpation.

Chest: No increased work of breathing. Mild cough noted.

Lungs: Breath sounds equal bilaterally. No wheezes, rhonchi, rales.

Heart: RRR. No murmurs noted. Peripheral pulses 2+ and equal.

Abdomen: Soft, non-tender, and non-distended. No hepatosplenomegaly noted.

Neurologic: A&O×3. No nuchal rigidity. Strength 5/5 for upper and lower extremities. DTR 2+ and equal bilaterally in the upper and lower extremities. Cranial nerves II to XII intact.

CLINICAL DISCUSSION QUESTIONS

1. What is the differential diagnosis?

_____

_____

_____

_____

2. What is the most likely diagnosis? Why?

_____

_____

_____

_____

3. Demonstrate your understanding about the pathophysiology in regard to the most likely diagnosis.

_____

_____

_____

_____

4. Should tests/imaging studies be ordered? Which ones? Why? Think about tests/imaging beyond the primary care setting as well.

_____

_____

_____

_____

5. What are the next appropriate steps in management?

_____

_____

_____

_____

6. Review credible research article(s) on this diagnosis. List your findings of the prevalence, preventive measures, and treatment options. Provide your reference(s).

_____

_____

_____

_____

7. What are the pertinent ICD-10 and CPT (E/M) codes for this visit? Provide a short rationale.

_____

_____

_____

_____

8. What is the appropriate patient education for this case?

_____

_____

_____

_____

9. If not managed appropriately, what is/are the medical/legal concern(s) that may arise?

_____

_____

_____

_____

10. Think about interprofessional collaboration for this case. Provide a list of specialties or other disciplines and indicate what contribution these professionals might make to managing the patient.

_____

_____

_____

_____

BEDSIDE MANNER QUESTIONS

11. What would your communication style/approach be with this patient and his mother?

_____

_____

_____

_____

12. If the patient and his mother are distressed by the diagnosis, what might offer support?

_____

_____

_____

_____

ANSWER KEY _available at_
https://connect.springerpub.com/content/book/978-0-8261-8273-9

BLURRY VISION, ADULT FEMALE

CHIEF COMPLAINT

"Blurry vision."

HISTORY OF PRESENT ILLNESS

A 32-year-old otherwise healthy woman presents to her PCP complaining of blurred vision, light-headedness, diplopia, and numbness in her lower extremities, tongue, and left side of her face. The symptoms became increasingly worse over a period of 2 months and then began to improve, with complete resolution of symptoms by the fourth month. The patient reported no relieving or aggravating factors while the symptoms were present.

REVIEW OF SYSTEMS

A ROS is positive for rash to anterior chest; occasional headache; double vision; blurred vision; numbness in lower extremities, tongue, and left side of face; and anxiety related to current symptoms. The ROS is negative for weight change, hearing loss, tinnitus, epistaxis, SOB, chest pain, cough, nausea, vomiting, diarrhea, abdominal pain, urinary symptoms, bruising, or temperature intolerance.

RELEVANT HISTORY

The patient's medical history is significant for measles at the age of 9 months and infectious mononucleosis at the age of 20. She wears glasses and contacts. Her family history is significant for hypertension in mother and father; her maternal grandfather has chronic renal failure. Her social history includes a 15-pack-year history of tobacco use, no alcohol, no illicit drug use. She lives with her husband and their golden retriever.

ALLERGIES

No known drug allergies; no known food allergies.

MEDICATIONS

None.

PHYSICAL EXAMINATION

Vitals: T 37.2°C (99.0°F), P 92, R 16, BP 122/72, WT 61.70 kg (136 lbs), HT 167.64 cm (66 in.), BMI 22.

General: Healthy appearing, well-dressed, well-groomed female in no apparent distress.

Skin, Hair, and Nails: Small and erythematous papules on the anterior chest under bilateral breasts. No abnormal findings with hair or nails.

Head: Atraumatic, normocephalic.

Eyes: EOM reveals a sixth nerve palsy of the left eye, decreased visual acuity of the right eye (OD 20/40) with an enlarged cup/disc ratio; PERRL.

Lungs: CTA bilaterally.

Heart: RRR; no murmurs, rubs, or gallops.

Lymphatic: No lymphadenopathy noted.

Neurologic: Positive Lhermitte sign; decreased sensation to L2 to L5 and S1 of lower extremities; DTR of bilateral lower extremities 1+ with decreased sensation of tongue and of the ophthalmic nerve distribution of the left side of the face.

CLINICAL DISCUSSION QUESTIONS

1. What is the differential diagnosis?

_____

_____

_____

_____

2. What is the most likely diagnosis? Why?

_____

_____

_____

_____

3. Demonstrate your understanding of the pathophysiology in regard to the most likely diagnosis.

_____

_____

_____

_____

4. Should tests/imaging studies be ordered? Which ones? Why? Think about tests/imaging beyond the primary care setting as well.

_____

_____

_____

_____

5. What are the next appropriate steps in management?

_____

_____

_____

_____

6. Review a recent and credible research article(s) about this diagnosis. Demonstrate your understanding of the diagnostic criteria, risk factors, and treatment options. Include a list of your reference(s).

_____

_____

_____

_____

7.   What are the pertinent ICD-10 and CPT (E/M) codes for this visit. Provide a short rationale.

_____

_____

_____

_____

8.   What is the appropriate patient education for this case?

_____

_____

_____

_____

9.   If not managed appropriately, what is/are the medical/legal concern(s) that may arise?

_____

_____

_____

_____

10.   Think about interprofessional collaboration for this case. Provide a list of specialties or other disciplines and indicate what contribution these professionals might make to managing the patient.

_____

_____

_____

_____

_____

BEDSIDE MANNER QUESTIONS

11.   What would your communication style/approach be with this patient?

_____

_____

_____

_____

12.   If a patient is distressed by the diagnosis, what might offer support?

_____

_____

_____

_____

ANSWER KEY *available at*
https://connect.springerpub.com/content/book/978-0-8261-8273-9

DOES NOT FOLLOW DIRECTIONS, PEDIATRIC MALE

CHIEF COMPLAINT

"Child does not follow directions."

HISTORY OF PRESENT ILLNESS

A mother brings her 8-year-old son to a PCP to evaluate his difficulty following directions. The mother states this has always been a problem at home and school; this year, his teacher is concerned as he is not completing in-class assignments. In addition, he makes careless mistakes on his work, is easily distracted, and loses things. He interrupts the teacher frequently and fidgets in his seat. He gets along well with other children and seems to want to obey the teacher but has a hard time remembering what he is to do. He has not received any detentions or suspensions and his mother states he is not a troublemaker at home or school.

REVIEW OF SYSTEMS

A ROS is negative for palpitations, SOB, and chest pain. No chronic cough or wheeze. No snoring or difficulty sleeping. No pruritus, allergic rhinitis, or eczema. No abdominal pain, diarrhea, constipation, vomiting. There is no history of anxiety, depression, or behavioral problems. No hospitalizations, chronic medical problems, or surgeries. The child sees a pediatric dentist every 6 months.

RELEVANT HISTORY

Tympanostomy tubes at 18 months and speech therapy for an expressive speech delay from 15 months until therapy ended at age 3. The boy was full-term, normal pregnancy. There is no maternal alcohol, drug, or nicotine use and the mother is G1P1. The child has no risk of exposure to lead. There is no family history of anxiety or depression. The boy's father struggled academically and was a "busy boy" in the classroom and at home. The family does not have a history of other mental illness or substance use or abuse or of cognitive delay or intellectual disability.

ALLERGIES

No known drug allergies; no known food allergies.

MEDICATIONS

None.

PHYSICAL EXAMINATION

Vitals: T 37°C (98.6°F), P 72, R 15, BP 107/66, HT 129.50 cm (51 in.), WT 24.95 kg (55 lbs), BMI 14.9.

General: Well-developed, well-nourished cooperative child in no acute distress. No atypical facies noted.

Skin, Hair, and Nails: No rashes or lesions noted.

Head: Normocephalic and atraumatic.

Eyes: PERRL; extraocular movements intact.

ENT/Mouth: TMs pearly gray, mobile. Clear nasal discharge. Posterior oropharynx clear with small amount of postnasal drip. Tonsils 2+ and equal bilaterally.

Neck: No cervical lymphadenopathy. No goiter noted.

Lungs: Clear to auscultation bilaterally; breath sounds equal.

Heart: RRR; no murmur noted.

Abdomen: Soft, non-tender, and non-distended.

Genital/Rectal: Sexual maturity rating stage 1; testicles descended bilaterally.

Neurologic: Cranial nerves II to XII grossly intact. Upper extremity and lower extremity strength 5/5 and equal bilaterally. Reflexes 2+ upper and lower extremities. Sensation normal upper and lower extremities. Gait is normal.

CLINICAL DISCUSSION QUESTIONS

1. What is the differential diagnosis?

_____

_____

_____

_____

2. What is the most likely diagnosis? Why?

_____

_____

_____

_____

3. Demonstrate your understanding about the pathophysiology in regard to the most likely diagnosis.

_____

_____

_____

_____

4. Should tests/imaging studies be ordered? Which ones? Why? Think about tests/imaging beyond the primary care setting as well.

_____

_____

_____

_____

5. What are the next appropriate steps in management?

_____

_____

_____

_____

6. What are the diagnostic criteria and treatment options for this diagnosis? Provide references for your response.

_____

_____

_____

_____

7. What are the pertinent ICD-10 and CPT (E/M) codes for this visit? Provide a short rationale.

_____

_____

_____

_____

8. What is the appropriate patient education for this case?

_____

_____

_____

_____

9. If not managed appropriately, what is/are the medical/legal concern(s) that may arise?

_____

_____

_____

_____

10. Think about interprofessional collaboration for this case. Provide a list of specialties or other disciplines and indicate what contribution these professionals might make to managing the patient.

_____

_____

_____

_____

BEDSIDE MANNER QUESTIONS

11. What would your communication style/approach be with this patient and his mother?

_____

_____

_____

_____

12. If a patient and his mother are distressed by the diagnosis, what might offer support?

_____

_____

_____

_____

ANSWER KEY *available at*
https://connect.springerpub.com/content/book/978-0-8261-8273-9

CRUSTY, IRRITATED LEFT EYE, PEDIATRIC MALE

CHIEF COMPLAINT

"Crusty, irritated left eye."

HISTORY OF PRESENT ILLNESS

A mother brings her 5-year-old son to his PCP with a complaint of a 3-day history of a "crusty and irritated" left eye. This morning the mother noticed increased erythema and crusty white drainage to the lashes and inner canthus. No medications or other treatments were given. The mother is wondering if it is pinkeye because the day care center the child attends after school notified parents yesterday there was a child diagnosed with it. The mother is requesting medication for the child to start treatment and asking if it is contagious and if she needs to take off at work to care for the child. She is concerned because she does not have the financial means to take off.

REVIEW OF SYSTEMS

A ROS is positive for left eye erythema and pruritus with white crusty drainage. The ROS is negative for pain or change in visual acuity, photosensitivity, or recent trauma. The mother denies the child has had a fever or change in appetite and energy. There is no ear pain, nasal congestion, sore throat, headache, cough, SOB, rash, or muscle aches. The mother denies a recent viral upper respiratory or ear infection. The mother denies any history of environmental or food allergies or history of allergic rhinitis.

RELEVANT HISTORY

There is no significant medical history of concern. The child is generally healthy and was a normal birth. The patient takes no routine medications. There have been no surgeries or hospitalizations. The family history is unremarkable. It is a nonsmoking home. The child lives with his mother and older brother. He attends kindergarten and an after-school day care program.

ALLERGIES

No known drug allergies; no known food allergies.

MEDICATIONS

None.

PHYSICAL EXAMINATION

Vitals: T 37°C (98.6°F), P 92, R 20, BP 106/54, WT 9.07 kg (46 lbs), HT 104.14 cm (41 in.), BMI 20.2.

General: The patient is in no apparent distress except for rubbing his eyes. He is acting appropriate for his age, is clean and dressed well, and has a caring mother at his side.

Psychiatric: Cooperative.

Skin, Hair, and Nails: Rest of the exam with no abnormal finding.

Head: Normocephalic.

Eyes: Left conjunctiva erythema with lid swelling and a small amount of yellow purulent drainage to the lashes. Right conjunctiva is normal. There is no visual acuity deficit. No foreign body. PERRL. Red reflex intact bilaterally.

Snellen Test: OD 20/20, OS 20/20, OU 20/20.

ENT/Mouth: TMs present bilaterally with no ear drainage or tenderness to palpation. There is no pre-auricular lymphadenopathy. Bilateral nares are without erythema, edema, or drainage. Oral mucosa is moist and normal. Normal dentation. Pharynx is normal.

Neck: No cervical lymphadenopathy. FROM.

Lungs: Clear to auscultation bilaterally.

Heart: RRR. No murmur.

Abdomen: BS present. Abdomen soft with no tenderness to palpation.

Musculoskeletal: Moves all extremities well with good strength.

Neurologic: Alert and oriented to person, place, and circumstance.

CLINICAL DISCUSSION QUESTIONS

1. What is the differential diagnosis?

_____

_____

_____

_____

2. What is the most likely diagnosis? Why?

_____

_____

_____

3. Demonstrate your understanding of the pathophysiology in regard to the most likely diagnosis.

_____

_____

_____

4. Should tests/imaging studies be ordered? Which ones? Why? Think about tests/imaging beyond the primary care setting as well.

_____

_____

_____

_____

5. What are the next appropriate steps in management?

_____

_____

_____

6. Review a recent and credible research article on making this diagnosis. Demonstrate your understanding of the treatment options and diagnostic criteria. Provide references.

_____

_____

_____

_____

7. What are the pertinent ICD-10 and CPT (E/M) codes for this visit? Provide a short rationale.

_____

_____

_____

_____

8. What is the appropriate patient education for this case?

_____

_____

_____

_____

9. If not managed appropriately, what is/are the medical/legal concern(s) that may arise?

_____

_____

_____

_____

10. Think about interprofessional collaboration for this case. Provide a list of specialties or other disciplines and indicate what contribution these professionals might make to managing the patient.

_____

_____

_____

_____

BEDSIDE MANNER QUESTIONS

11. What would your communication style/approach be with this patient and his mother?

_____

_____

_____

_____

12. If a patient and his mother are distressed by the diagnosis, what might offer support?

_____

_____

_____

_____

ANSWER KEY _available at_
https://connect.springerpub.com/content/book/978-0-8261-8273-9

FREQUENT URINATION, ADULT MALE

CHIEF COMPLAINT

"Frequent urination."

HISTORY OF PRESENT ILLNESS

A 42-year-old man with a history of hypertension and substance use disorder comes to the primary care clinic for a mandatory health checkup. He is on court probation and living in a sober house that requires an intake physical. He complains of fatigue, frequent urination, excessive thirst, and blurred vision. He also reports gradual weight gain and tingling and numbness in his extremities, which make performing chores in the sober house difficult. His symptoms started about 2 years ago but have never been checked as he has been in and out of jail. His urination frequency and the volume output are getting worse. He reports seeing ants around the toilet bowl every morning for about 2 weeks. He drinks a lot of water (about half gallon daily), but there been has no improvement. He was concerned about these symptoms because his older brother was diagnosed with diabetes and both parents had died from complications of diabetes. He used cocaine to relax and not worry about his symptoms.

REVIEW OF SYSTEMS

A ROS is positive for the symptoms related in the HPI: polyuria, polydipsia, paresthesia, blurred vision, fatigue, and weight gain. The patient reports dry skin, cuts, and bruises that are slow to heal, poor dentition, and abdominal bloating. He reports cravings and feeling down but denies significant opioid withdrawal symptoms. The ROS is negative for fever, chills, headaches, diarrhea, or vomiting. He denies any blood in the urine, dysuria, or urge incontinence and has no known history of sexually transmitted diseases. He has no chest pain, stomachache, backache, extremity pain, or edema.

RELEVANT HISTORY

The patient has a medical history of hypertension (diagnosed 5 years prior but is not on antihypertensives when he comes to the clinic). He also has a history of substance use disorder involving inhaled cocaine and occasional intravenous heroin use. He had recently seen a behavioral health specialist at the sober house. He has no history of surgery or hospitalization. Both parents died in their early 60s from complications of diabetes. An older brother was diagnosed with type 2 diabetes at age 42 and prostate cancer at age 50. His younger sister is in good health. Since graduating from high school, he has worked as a truck driver, transporting alcoholic beverages from Connecticut to Florida. He is planning to resume this job after completing his court probation. He is divorced and has two adult sons; both are in good health. For a long time, he depended on fast foods and never had time to exercise. He uses alcohol socially and smokes half a pack per day. He is unemployed and uninsured and has no support system except for the counselors at the sober house.

ALLERGIES

No known drug allergies; no known food allergies.

MEDICATIONS

Methadone (50 mg daily); directly observed therapy at the methadone clinic.

PHYSICAL EXAMINATION

Vitals: T 37°C (98.6°F), P 80, R 14, BP 150/88, WT 109 kg (240.3 lbs), HT 175 cm (68.9 in.), waist circumference 42 in., BMI 35.6.

General: Well-developed and -nourished middle-aged African American man in no acute distress.

Psychiatric: Mildly anxious with a flat affect.

Skin, Hair, and Nails: Skin dry with discoloration in body folds, no rashes, or bleeding tendency. Hair intact. Nails yellow and brittle.

Head: Normocephalic.

Eyes: Vision reduced bilaterally; pupils equal and reactive to light. Intraretinal hemorrhages, exudates, and cotton wool spots in both eyes.

ENT/Mouth: Tympanic membrane pearly, grey with no fluid. Oral mucosa moist; dentition in bad repair with easy gum bleeding.

Neck: Supple with no adenopathy or thyroid enlargement.

Chest: No deformities noted.

Lungs: Clear to auscultation bilaterally.

Breasts: Non-tender; no lumps.

Heart: RRR, without murmur, gallop, or rubs.

Peripheral Vascular: Faint dorsalis pedis and posterior tibial pulses (1/4).

Abdomen: Soft with no masses, organomegaly, or tenderness. Active bowel sounds in all four quadrants.

Genital/Rectal: No penile or testicular abnormalities noted. Prostate within normal limits.

Lymphatics: No axillary or inguinal lymphadenopathy.

Musculoskeletal: No deformities, tenderness, or edema. Full range of motion in all joints.

Neurologic: A&O×3; cranial nerves II to XII grossly intact. Reflexes present in all extremities. Mild defects on proprioception, vibration, and monofilament sensation.

Point-of-Care Testing: Point-of-care laboratory testing revealed a random blood glucose of 340 mg/dL, 3+ glucose in urine, and no ketones. HbA1C was 8.8%.

CLINICAL DISCUSSION QUESTIONS

1. What is the differential diagnosis?

_____

_____

_____

_____

2. What is the most likely diagnosis? Why?

_____

_____

_____

_____

3. Demonstrate your understanding about the pathophysiology in regard to the most likely diagnosis.

_____

_____

_____

_____

4. Should tests/imaging studies be ordered? Which ones? Why? Think about tests/imaging beyond the primary care setting as well.

_____

_____

_____

_____

5. What are the next appropriate steps in management?

_____

_____

_____

6. Review a recent and credible research article(s) about this diagnosis. Demonstrate your understanding of the prevalence, diagnostic criteria, and treatment options. Include a list of reference(s).

_____

_____

_____

_____

7. What are the pertinent ICD-10 and CPT (E/M) codes for this visit? Provide a short rationale.

_____

_____

_____

_____

8. What are the appropriate patient education topics for this case?

_____

_____

_____

_____

9. If not managed appropriately, what is/are the medical/legal concern(s) that may arise?

_____

_____

_____

_____

10. Think about interprofessional collaboration for this case. Provide a list of specialties or other disciplines and indicate what contribution these professionals might make to managing the patient.

_____

_____

_____

BEDSIDE MANNER QUESTIONS

11. What would your communication style/approach be with this patient?

_____

_____

_____

_____

12. If a patient is distressed by the diagnosis, what might offer support?

_____

_____

_____

_____

ANSWER KEY _available at_
https://connect.springerpub.com/content/book/978-0-8261-8273-9

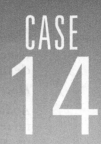

VOMITING, PEDIATRIC MALE

CHIEF COMPLAINT
"Vomiting."

HISTORY OF PRESENT ILLNESS
A mother brings her 7-year-old fully immunized and previously well son for an evaluation of his vomiting for the past 2 days. The mother reports the child is unable to tolerate any oral intake, including fluids, and she is concerned about dehydration. She states he has been fatigued and sleepy appearing as of today. The boy states he is thirsty and has been urinating more often but denies diarrhea, abdominal pain, dysuria, constipation, hematochezia, hematuria, or consumption of unsafe foods. His last bowel movement this morning was normal. His mother denies fevers, recent travel, drinking from streams/wells, and meeting with known sick contacts.

REVIEW OF SYSTEMS
The child's ROS is positive for nausea, vomiting, fatigue, unintentional weight loss, frequent urination, polydipsia, and inability to tolerate fluids. His ROS is negative for fevers, chills, sore throat, rhinorrhea, cough, SOB, chest pain, abdominal pain, diarrhea, constipation, hematochezia, melena, passage of worms, dysuria, hematuria, testicular pain, groin pain, polyphagia, myalgias, arthralgias, and delayed growth/small for stature.

RELEVANT HISTORY
The patient's immunizations are up to date. The boy was a full-term birth without complications, and he has had no prior medical problems. He lives with his parents and sister in a single-family home. He eats a well-balanced diet and limits sugary beverages and foods. His family history is significant for Graves disease in his mother and lupus as well as Sjogren syndrome in his maternal grandmother. All other first-line relatives are well and healthy.

ALLERGIES
No known drug allergies; no known food allergies.

MEDICATIONS
None.

PHYSICAL EXAMINATION
Vitals: T 36.9°C (98.4°F); P 112; R 20; BP 102/62; HT 122 cm (48 in.); 50th percentile, WT 21 kg (46 lbs); 25th percentile, BMI 14; 10th percentile, POCBG "high."

General: Alert, nontoxic, appearing tired.

Skin, Hair, and Nails: Dry, pale, decreased skin turgor, no jaundice. No abnormal findings with hair. Delayed capillary refill at 3 sec, no clubbing.

Head: Normocephalic/atraumatic.

Eyes: Appearing sunken in.

Mouth/ENT: Dry mucous membranes, no lesions, uvula midline, no oropharyngeal erythema, no tonsillar swelling/exudate.

Neck: No lymphadenopathy, no thyromegaly or masses.

Breasts: No gynecomastia.

Lungs: Clear to auscultation bilaterally, mild Kussmaul breathing, no retractions or accessory muscle use.

Heart: RRR; no murmurs, rubs, or gallops.

Abdomen: Non-distended; bowel sounds present; soft, mild generalized tenderness to palpation; no rebound; no guarding; non-tender McBurney point; negative Murphy sign; negative psoas sign; negative Rovsing sign; negative obturator sign; negative jarring tenderness; no peritoneal signs; no hepatosplenomegaly.

Genital: Circumcised male; no penile lesions, erythema, or discharge; no scrotal swelling or erythema; bilateral testes in proper position, non-tender.

Neurologic: Answers questions appropriately, no focal neurologic deficits.

CLINICAL DISCUSSION QUESTIONS

1. What is the differential diagnosis?

_____

_____

_____

2. What is the most likely diagnosis? Why?

_____

_____

_____

3. Demonstrate your understanding about the pathophysiology in regard to the most likely diagnosis.

_____

_____

_____

4. Should tests/imaging studies be ordered? Which ones? Why? Think about tests/imaging beyond the primary care setting as well.

_____

_____

_____

5. What are the next appropriate steps in management?

_____

_____

_____

6. How does this medical condition in a child adversely affect an entire family? Provide references for your response.

_____

_____

_____

_____

7. What are the pertinent ICD-10 and CPT (E/M) codes for this visit? Provide a short rationale.

_____

_____

_____

_____

8. What is the appropriate patient/parent education for this case?

_____

_____

_____

_____

9. If not managed appropriately, what is/are the medical/legal concern(s) that may arise?

_____

_____

_____

_____

10. Think about interprofessional collaboration for this case. Provide a list of specialties or other disciplines and indicate what contribution these professionals might make to managing the patient.

_____

_____

_____

_____

BEDSIDE MANNER QUESTION

11. What would your communication style/approach be with this parent and patient?

_____

_____

_____

_____

ANSWER KEY _available at_
https://connect.springerpub.com/content/book/978-0-8261-8273-9

DIFFICULTY RELATING TO OTHERS, PEDIATRIC MALE

CHIEF COMPLAINT

"Difficulty relating to others."

HISTORY OF PRESENT ILLNESS

A mother brings her 4-year-old son to their PCP to address his difficulties at home and school over the past 2 months. His pre-school teacher requested a meeting last week and reported to the mother that her son seems to not pay attention during class. He stares off and often does not answer or make eye contact with her when she asks a question. The teacher also said he often stands up during class and walks around the room, disturbing his classmates. During group activities, he often gets upset with peers and repeats "doing it wrong" until he is allowed to finish the task alone. Despite all of this, he demonstrates mastery of the material. The mother explains her son does not look her in the eyes much either, or she often needs to say something a few times before he responds. He had been receiving early intervention speech therapy and occupational therapy since he was 15 months old. She states the interventions helped and were discontinued at age 2, but he continued some behaviors that have now worsened. He has never really been interested in playing with his siblings, but now he gets upset and cries if they try to play with him. The mother states he would spend hours playing with his toy cars if she let him, putting them in rows and then back in their containers. She has noticed he is picky about food. A speech therapist was able to get him to eat a few new foods, but now most days he only wants chicken nuggets and mashed potatoes. Overall, his mother's main concern is his ability to continue in school and make some friends.

REVIEW OF SYSTEMS

A ROS is positive for changes in appetite and mood. All other symptoms are negative.

RELEVANT HISTORY

The child's medical history is significant for speech and fine motor delays diagnosed at 13 months. He received speech and occupational therapy from age 15 months to 24 months. He was a full-term baby and the pregnancy was uncomplicated. All newborn screenings were normal. The child has had no significant illnesses and is up to date on immunizations.

The child lives with his parents and two siblings (ages 5 and 9). He sleeps 8 hours a night and often takes a 1-hour afternoon nap. He attends a half day of pre-school in the morning. His mother works part-time in the morning while he is at school but is otherwise home with him. He sits in a booster seat in the car and wears a helmet when riding his bicycle. There are no firearms in the house or no second-hand smoke exposure. There is no significant family history.

ALLERGIES

No known drug allergies; no known food allergies.

MEDICATIONS

Daily multivitamin.

PHYSICAL EXAMINATION

Vitals: T 37°C (98.6°F), P 82, R 18, BP 92/58, WT 18 kg (39.7 lbs), HT 101.5 cm (39.75 in.), BMI 17.5.

General: No acute distress but agitated during exam, sitting quietly next to mother playing with toy car.

Psychiatric: Complies with exam but disinterested, answers questions with short responses, little eye contact with mother or provider, spinning/examining wheels of toy car repetitively throughout exam.

Skin, Hair, and Nails: Skin warm and dry; no rashes, lesions, bruising, or discoloration.

Head: Normocephalic and atraumatic.

Eyes: PERRLA; extraocular eye movements intact.

ENT/Mouth: Ear canal clear, tympanic membranes visible bilaterally without erythema or effusion, nares patent, turbinates pink and moist, good oral hygiene, oropharynx mucosa pink and moist.

Neck: No masses, no lymphadenopathy.

Lungs: Clear to auscultation bilaterally.

Heart: RRR, no murmurs.

Abdomen: Bowel sounds active, soft, non-tender, non-distended.

Musculoskeletal: Strength 5/5 upper and lower extremities.

Neurologic: Cranial nerves II to XII grossly intact, good muscle tone.

CLINICAL DISCUSSION QUESTIONS

1. What is the differential diagnosis?

_____

_____

_____

_____

2. What is the most likely diagnosis? Why?

_____

_____

_____

_____

3. Demonstrate your understanding about the pathophysiology in regard to the most likely diagnosis.

_____

_____

_____

_____

4. Should tests/imaging studies be ordered? Which ones? Why? Think about tests/imaging beyond the primary care setting as well.

_____

_____

_____

_____

5. What is the next appropriate step in management?

_____

_____

_____

_____

6. According to the most recent research, what are the key factors in making the diagnosis and the prevalence of the diagnosis? Provide references for your response.

_____

_____

_____

_____

7. What are the pertinent ICD-10 and CPT (E/M) codes for this visit? Provide a short rationale.

_____

_____

_____

_____

8. What are the appropriate patient education topics for this case?

_____

_____

_____

_____

9. If not managed appropriately, what is/are the medical/legal concern(s) that may arise?

_____

_____

_____

_____

10. Think about interprofessional collaboration for this case. Provide a list of specialties or other disciplines and indicate what contribution these professionals might make to managing the patient?

_____

_____

_____

_____

BEDSIDE MANNER QUESTIONS

11. What would your communication style/approach be with this patient's mother?

_____

_____

_____

_____

12. If a patient's mother is distressed by the diagnosis, what might offer support?

_____

_____

_____

_____

ANSWER KEY *available at*
https://connect.springerpub.com/content/book/978-0-8261-8273-9

FACIAL NUMBNESS, ADULT MALE

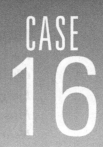

CHIEF COMPLAINT

"Facial numbness."

HISTORY OF PRESENT ILLNESS

A 38-year-old previously well man presents complaining of new onset left-sided facial droop and numbness upon waking this morning. The patient reports drooling, particularly while drinking or eating, and states his morning coffee tasted "weird." He denies any sick contacts, recent illnesses, history of the same, pain, head trauma, fever, headache, extremity weakness, confusion, anxiousness, abnormal speech, and vision changes, although he notes that his left eye is dry because it is difficult to shut it. The patient admits to a history of hypertension, hyperlipidemia, and tobacco use but states compliance with his medications as well as recent attempts at tobacco cessation (reducing from 0.5 pack per day to approximately 5 cigarettes per day). He reports use of over-the-counter lubricating drops for his left eye to alleviate the dryness. He denies any other therapy. He attempted to make an appointment with his regular PCP but is unable to be seen there until next month, so he presents now to the urgent care clinic affiliated with the PCP's practice.

REVIEW OF SYSTEMS

The patient's ROS is positive for unilateral facial muscle weakness, facial numbness, an inability to close the left eyelid, dry eye, drooling, and taste changes. ROS is negative for fever, pain, trauma, headache, vision changes, confusion, anxiousness, extremity weakness/numbness/tingling, seizures, and dysphasia.

RELEVANT HISTORY

The patient's medical history is significant for hypertension (diagnosed 15 years ago and well controlled), hyperlipidemia (compliant on statins for 10 years), and obesity. His social history is pertinent for tobacco use (20-pack-year history). The family history is noncontributory.

ALLERGIES

Penicillin (reaction: hives); no known food allergies.

MEDICATIONS

- Hydrochlorothiazide 12.5 mg, 1 tablet PO QD.
- Simvastatin, 20 mg, 1 tablet PO QHS.

PHYSICAL EXAMINATION

Vitals: T 36.9°C (98.4°F), P 77, R 16, BP 116/76 mmHg, HT 178 cm (70 in.), WT 109.8 kg (242 lbs), BMI 34.7

General: A&O×4. Nontoxic appearing. Ambulates with steady gait. Speaks in full sentences.

Psychiatric: Cooperative.

Head: Normocephalic/atraumatic. +Facial asymmetry. No left forehead creases with raising of eyebrows.

Eyes: Left ptosis. Left mild scleral injection. PERRL bilaterally. EOM intact bilaterally. Conjunctivae pink bilaterally. Non-tender to palpation bilaterally.

Mouth: Left droop, drooling. Moist mucous membranes.

Neck: FROM.

Chest: RRR. No murmurs, rubs, or gallops.

Lungs: Clear to auscultation bilaterally. Unlabored respiration.

Musculoskeletal: 5/5 equal strengths in all extremities. Sensation grossly intact.

Neurologic: Left-sided facial droop. Cranial nerves III/V/VII decreased. Decreased sharp/dull sensation to left side of face. No (dysphasia) slurred speech. No pronator drift. Cranial nerves II, IV, VI, IX to XII intact.

CLINICAL DISCUSSION QUESTIONS

1. What is the differential diagnosis?

_____

_____

_____

_____

2. What is the most likely diagnosis? Why?

_____

_____

_____

_____

3. Demonstrate your understanding about the pathophysiology in regard to the most likely diagnosis.

_____

_____

_____

_____

4. Should tests/imaging studies be ordered? Which ones? Why? Think about tests/imaging beyond the primary care setting as well.

_____

_____

_____

_____

5. What are the next appropriate steps in management?

_____

_____

_____

_____

6. Review a recent and credible research article(s) about this diagnosis. Demonstrate your understanding of the diagnostic testing, prognosis, and treatment plan. Include a list of your reference(s).

_____

_____

_____

_____

7. What are the pertinent ICD-10 and CPT (E/M) codes for this visit? Provide a short rationale.

_____

_____

_____

_____

8. What is the appropriate patient education for this case?

_____

_____

_____

_____

9. If not managed appropriately, what is/are the medical/legal concern(s) that may arise?

_____

_____

_____

_____

10. Think about interprofessional collaboration for this case. Provide a list of specialties or other disciplines and indicate what contribution these professionals might make to managing the patient?

_____

_____

_____

_____

BEDSIDE MANNER QUESTIONS

11. What would your communication style/approach be with this patient?

_____

_____

_____

_____

12. If the patient is distressed by the diagnosis, what might offer support?

_____

_____

_____

_____

ANSWER KEY _available at_
https://connect.springerpub.com/content/book/978-0-8261-8273-9

ELBOW INJURY, PEDIATRIC MALE

CHIEF COMPLAINT

"Elbow injury."

HISTORY OF PRESENT ILLNESS

A mother brings her 5-year-old son to his PCP for a follow-up after an urgent care visit 2 days ago. His mother took him to urgent care after he complained of left elbow pain and had stopped using the arm. The mother states the elbow pain began after a fall earlier that day. She said he had been running around the house and she told him he needed to slow down or he would hurt himself; he then fell forward and hit his left elbow. When asked about the injury, the patient said, "I hurt my elbow. Mom got mad because I was running so much." The mother states she thinks he hurt his back too when he fell, but otherwise there were no other injuries. He had an x-ray at the urgent care. The mother states there were no fractures, but the physician in the urgent care recommended a follow-up because the boy had dislocated his elbow. Mother did not bring the radiology report for the PCP to review. He has been doing well with icing his arm, taking ibuprofen 150 mg TID, and resting his arm. He said there is less pain today, but he is afraid to use his arm.

REVIEW OF SYSTEMS

The ROS is positive for left elbow pain, low back pain, and bruising on the lower back. There is no head injury, joint swelling, numbness, weakness, or paresthesia of upper or lower extremities. All other symptoms are negative.

RELEVANT HISTORY

The boy's medical history is significant for a second-degree burn on the right anterior thigh 3 months prior from a curling iron that fell off counter. There are no other significant medical history or injuries. The child lives with both parents and a grandmother, who has Alzheimer's disease. He sleeps 10 hours per night. He is in kindergarten and states he does not really like school. His mother stated he was doing well but now "doesn't do everything he should be doing for school." The child always wears the seat belt in the car and a helmet when riding his bicycle. No second-hand smoke exposure, firearms in the house, or significant family history were reported.

ALLERGIES

No known drug or food allergies.

MEDICATIONS

None.

PHYSICAL EXAMINATION

Vitals: T 37°C (98.6°F), P 100, R 20, BP 98/62, WT 18 kg (39.68 lbs), HT 108 cm (42.5 in.), BMI 15.4.

General: Well-dressed/well-groomed, guarding left arm, mother close by during the entire exam.

Psychiatric: Engaged during the exam and between questions and exam with a downward gaze; appears anxious and withdrawn when compared to smiling and talkative baseline from previous PCP visits.

Skin, Hair, and Nails: Skin warm and dry, no rashes; well-healed scar on right anterior thigh; mild swelling, but no bruising or warmth over the left elbow; four linear bruises each 15 cm × 2 cm on buttocks in various stages of healing. No other bruises or lesions. Hair and nails showed no abnormal findings.

Head: Normocephalic, non-tender, and atraumatic.

Lungs: Clear to auscultation bilaterally.

Heart: RRR; no murmurs; brisk capillary refill; no cyanosis; distal pulses intact, upper and lower extremities.

Abdomen: Bowel sounds active in all quadrants, soft, non-tender, non-distended.

Neurological: Sensation intact and equal bilaterally for upper and lower extremities; no spinal tenderness.

Musculoskeletal: Mild tenderness of lateral left forearm; no focal tenderness of elbow. Refuses active range of motion, full passive range of motion left elbow. Full active and passive range of motion right elbow and bilateral fingers, wrists, and shoulders.

CLINICAL DISCUSSION QUESTIONS

1. What is the differential diagnosis?

_____

_____

_____

_____

2. What is the most likely diagnosis? Why?

_____

_____

_____

_____

3. Demonstrate your understanding about the pathophysiology in regard to the most likely diagnosis.

_____

_____

_____

_____

4. Should tests/imaging studies be ordered? Which ones? Why? Think about tests/imaging beyond the primary care setting as well.

_____

_____

_____

_____

5. What are the next appropriate steps in management?

_____

_____

_____

_____

6. Review a recent and credible research article(s) about this diagnosis. Demonstrate your understanding of the prevalence, risk factors, and treatment approach. Include a list of your reference(s).

_____

_____

_____

_____

7. What are the pertinent ICD-10 and CPT (E/M) codes for this visit? Provide a short rationale.

_____

_____

_____

_____

8. What are the appropriate patient and parent education topics for this case?

_____

_____

_____

_____

9. If not managed appropriately, what is/are the medical/legal concern(s) that may arise?

_____

_____

_____

_____

10. Think about interprofessional collaboration for this case. Provide a list of specialties or other disciplines and indicate what contribution these professionals might make to managing the patient.

_____

_____

_____

_____

BEDSIDE MANNER QUESTION

11. What would your communication style/approach be with this patient and his mother?

_____

_____

_____

_____

ANSWER KEY *available at*
https://connect.springerpub.com/content/book/978-0-8261-8273-9

THICK YELLOW TOENAILS, ADULT FEMALE

CHIEF COMPLAINT

"Thick, yellow toenails."

HISTORY OF PRESENT ILLNESS

A 64-year-old woman presents for her monthly check-in appointment. She has several chronic conditions that are well controlled through medications, and she follows up with specialists involved in her care every 6 months. She is having surgery for a right rotator cuff tear later in the month and would like to discuss her thick, discolored toenails. She has had a number of health problems in the past 5 years requiring medication adjustments and surgeries, and she believes she is "caught up" enough to get something done about her toenails. She reports her nails are very thick ("I haven't been able to cut my nails in years"), curled, and yellow. She saw a podiatrist about her hammertoe surgical repair last year, but she did not mention her toenails. She remembers having very "pretty" toenails in her 20s and 30s. She would wear nail polish but stopped at least 20 years ago. She has never injured her toenails, never wore high heels, and does not remember ever having a fungal infection.

REVIEW OF SYSTEMS

The patient's ROS is positive for toenail discoloration and malformation. She denies rash or skin lesions on feet, limping, numbness, or tingling.

RELEVANT HISTORY

The patient's medical history is significant for diabetes mellitus type 2, controlled with insulin and diet, and bilateral hammertoe of the great toes. Her surgical history includes a right carpal tunnel repair, bilateral bunionectomies, right shoulder rotator cuff repair, right trigger finger release, left shoulder arthroscopy, and right shoulder repair. She has a long history of chronic pain from rheumatoid arthritis and cervical and lumbar disc herniation, for which she is stable on chronic narcotics. The patient is married and on long-term disability because of multiple health problems. She is sexually active and lives with her husband and a roommate. Her exercise is a daily walk, using a walker, to the end of the driveway. Her family history is unknown as she was adopted as a toddler.

ALLERGIES

No known drug or food allergies.

MEDICATIONS

- Lantus 100 units/mL solution, Sig: 60 units at bedtime nightly.
- Oxycodone hydrochloride 15 mg tablet, Sig: 1 tab PO q6h PRN for pain.
- Sotalol 80 mg tablet, Sig: one tab PO BID.
- Rosuvastatin calcium 40 mg tablet, Sig: 1 tab PO QD.
- Citalopram 60 mg tablet, Sig: 1 tablet PO QD.
- Amlodipine 5 mg tablet, Sig: 1 tab PO QD.
- Linagliptin 5 mg tablet, Sig: 1 tab PO QD.
- Aspirin enteric coated 81 mg delayed-release tablet, Sig: 1 tab PO QD

PHYSICAL EXAMINATION

Vitals: T 37°C (98.6°F), P 73, R 16, BP 118/72, HT 171.45 cm (67.5 in.), WT 120.6 kg (266 lbs), BMI 41.04.

General: Well-appearing woman, no acute distress, appears stated age, sitting comfortably in chair. Front-wheeled walker near chair.

Psychiatric: Mildly anxious.

Skin, Hair, and Nails: Skin normal in appearance; no rashes or lesions. Normal hair distribution, thin on top of scalp. Fingernails normal in color, texture, and shape; neatly trimmed to edge of nail bed, no cyanosis/clubbing. Toenails on bilateral feet deep yellow, thickened, and curved inward, extending beyond edge of toe.

Head: Normal shape and appearance.

Lungs: Clear in all lobes.

Heart: RRR without murmur.

Neurologic: A&O×3; color, sensation, and movement within normal limits on bilateral legs and feet.

CLINICAL DISCUSSION QUESTIONS

1. What is the differential diagnosis?

2. What is the most likely diagnosis? Why?

3. Demonstrate your understanding of the pathophysiology in regard to the most likely diagnosis.

4. Should tests/imaging studies be ordered? Which ones? Why? Think about tests/imaging beyond the primary care setting as well.

5. What are the next appropriate steps in management?

_____

_____

_____

_____

6. Review a credible research article(s) about this diagnosis. Demonstrate your understanding of the prevalence, diagnostic criteria, and treatment options. Include a list of your reference(s).

_____

_____

_____

_____

7. What are the pertinent ICD-10 and CPT (E/M) codes for this visit? Provide a short rationale.

_____

_____

_____

_____

8. What are the appropriate patient education topics for this case?

_____

_____

_____

_____

9. If not managed appropriately, what is/are the medical/legal concern(s) that may arise?

_____

_____

_____

_____

10. Think about interprofessional collaboration for this case. Provide a list of specialties or other disciplines and indicate what contribution these professionals might make to managing the patient.

_____

_____

_____

_____

BEDSIDE MANNER QUESTION

11. What would your communication style/approach be with this patient?

_____

_____

_____

_____

ANSWER KEY *available at*
https://connect.springerpub.com/content/book/978-0-8261-8273-9

SPEECH DIFFICULTIES, GERIATRIC MALE

CHIEF COMPLAINT
"Speech difficulties."

HISTORY OF PRESENT ILLNESS
A 74-year-old man, accompanied by his son, presents for evaluation of speech changes over the past 6 months. The patient denies significant change in voice, but his son provides history that his father's voice has grown softer, speech is now slowly produced, and it is difficult to understand him at times. This has made communication over the phone particularly challenging. The patient's son lives out of state, so he had not seen his father in person for about 8 months and they rely on phone communication. The son states he was a bit surprised upon seeing his dad because he noted not only the voice and speech-pattern changes but also a tremor in his right hand. The patient denies experiencing any falls in the last year.

REVIEW OF SYSTEMS
A ROS is positive for skin dryness, increasingly vivid dreams, and tremor in the right hand. The patient's ROS is negative for anxiety, depression, weight loss, or fatigue. No recent or other trauma stated. He is negative for head injuries recently or in the past. No numbness, tingling, or paresthesia in the hand(s) noted.

MEDICAL HISTORY
The patient denies use of prescription medications or chronic medical conditions. He takes a men's daily multivitamin but no other supplements. His social history includes one 3-ounce-serving of whiskey each night before bed. Alcohol does not seem to affect the tremor. He was a tobacco smoker, 1 pack per day for 15 years but quit 25 years ago. He denies illicit drug use now or in the past. He denies exposure to neurotoxins or other chemicals. His family history includes mother, deceased, at age 94, natural causes; father, deceased, at 56, motor vehicle accident; a younger sister, 68, with hyperthyroid and depression, which are managed; one adult son, an adult daughter, and three granddaughters, all healthy. He was widowed 3 years ago. He denies any family history of tremor.

ALLERGIES
Penicillin (hives); no known food allergies.

MEDICATIONS
Men's daily multivitamin, generic.

PHYSICAL EXAMINATION

Vitals: T 37°C (98.6°F), P 78, R 22, BP: 110/78, HT: 182.88 cm (72 in.); WT: 80.28 kg (177 lbs); BMI 24.

General: Well nourished, good hygiene, no acute distress, decreased spontaneous facial expressions.

Psychiatric: Able to follow commands, cooperative with physical exam, slow to answer history questions.

Skin, Hair, and Nails: Seborrheic dermatitis present around the nasal labial folds and eyebrows.

ENT/Mouth: Voice quality poor (low volume); speech lacks spontaneity and fluidity when produced; extraocular movements intact in six cardinal positions of gaze.

Musculoskeletal: 5/5 strength in bilateral upper and lower extremities; no atrophy of musculature or reduced range of motion.

Neurologic: DTRs 2+ equal and symmetrical in bilateral upper and lower extremities; positive for glabellar reflex; no increased tone through passive motion in left upper extremity or bilateral lower extremities; right upper extremity exhibits cogwheeling at the wrist and elbow that worsens with distraction; supination-pronation tremor noted at rest in the right hand; slight jaw tremor noted; gait/balance assessment: patient needed three attempts to rise from the chair using hands, positive retropulsion test, shuffling gait present with reduced stride length; reduced arm swing in the right arm on ambulation; negative Romberg sensation intact to light and sharp touch on plantar surfaces of feet bilaterally; writing assessment: handwriting is small and illegible, impaired ability to copy a spiral (patient's rendition appears smaller with less fluid lines compared to provider's example); rapid alternating movements impaired in the right upper extremity; Mini-Mental State Exam score = 26/30.

CLINICAL DISCUSSION QUESTIONS

1. What is the differential diagnosis?

_____

_____

_____

_____

2. What is the most likely diagnosis? Why?

_____

_____

_____

_____

3. Demonstrate your understanding about the pathophysiology in regard to the most likely diagnosis.

_____

_____

_____

_____

4. Should tests/imaging studies be ordered? Which ones? Why? Think about tests/imaging beyond the primary care setting as well.

_____

_____

_____

_____

5. What are the next appropriate steps in management?

_____

_____

_____

_____

6. What are the clinical presentations, diagnostic criteria, and treatment approaches for this diagnosis? Provide references for your response.

_____

_____

_____

_____

7. What are the pertinent ICD-10 and CPT (E/M) codes for this visit? Provide a short rationale.

_____

_____

_____

_____

8. What is the appropriate patient education for this case?

_____

_____

_____

_____

9. If not managed appropriately, what is/are the medical/legal concern(s) that may arise?

_____

_____

_____

_____

10. Think about interprofessional collaboration for this case. Provide a list of specialties or other disciplines and indicate what contribution these professionals might make to managing the patient.

_____

_____

_____

_____

BEDSIDE MANNER QUESTIONS

11. What would your communication style/approach be with this patient and his son?

_____

_____

_____

_____

12. If a patient and his son are distressed by the diagnosis, what might offer support?

_____

_____

_____

_____

ANSWER KEY _available at_
https://connect.springerpub.com/content/book/978-0-8261-8273-9

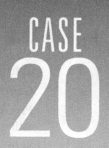

MOOD CHANGES, ADULT MALE

CHIEF COMPLAINT
"Mood changes."

HISTORY OF PRESENT ILLNESS
A 34-year-old man presents to a primary care office for evaluation of mood changes. He says he has been more easily agitated and his partner has noted an increase in irritability. His husband has asked him to be evaluated for depression. He has been treated for depression in the past. He denies current symptoms of depression but says he has been fatigued in the past year and has suffered frequent headaches. Despite exercising regularly, he has had weight gain, daytime fatigue, and joint pain.

His husband has also asked that he sleep in another room because of his snoring. He had been using a CPAP machine for obstructive sleep apnea but finds the head strap increasingly uncomfortable to wear because of how tight it is despite attempts to adjust it. For this reason, he often does not use it. The patient recently had blood work done as part of a routine physical 3 weeks ago that found he was "pre-diabetic" and had elevated cholesterol.

He is also upset because he has stopped wearing his wedding ring and a watch that was his father's because they are now too small for him. He attributes this to the weight gain despite a healthy diet and regular exercise.

REVIEW OF SYSTEMS
The patient's ROS is positive for worsening peripheral vision, excessive sweating, fatigue, weight gain, headaches, sleep difficulties, change in mood, erectile dysfunction, skin darkening (around neck and axilla), and joint pain.

The ROS is negative for bowel or bladder dysfunction, suicidal/homicidal ideation, head injury, change in appetite or thirst, seizures, loss of consciousness, numbness or tingling, involuntary movements or spasms, and abdominal pain.

RELEVANT HISTORY
The patient's medical history is significant for obstructive sleep apnea, not controlled; hypertension; osteoarthritis of the right knee; newly diagnosed pre-diabetes and hypercholesterolemia, which that he is attempting to manage with lifestyle modifications. The patient denies alcohol, tobacco, or illicit drug use now or in the past. He has been married to the same man for 6 years; no children, no siblings.

ALLERGIES
No known drug allergies; no known food allergies.

MEDICATIONS
- Hydrochlorothiazide 12.5 mg PO QD.
- Acetaminophen 1,000 mg PO QID PRN for knee pain.

PHYSICAL EXAMINATION

Vitals: T 37.5°C (99.5°F), P 82, R 18, BP 142/86 mmHg, HT 190.5 cm (75 in.), WT 108.86 kg (240 lbs), BMI 31.

General: Well developed, well nourished, no acute distress.

Psychiatric: Able to maintain attention and answer questions; PHQ-9 score 6 (mild depression, affirmative answers only to "feeling tired" and "trouble staying asleep").

Skin, Hair, and Nails: Dense facial hair distribution, velvety darkening of the skin around the neck and axilla; skin is moist diffusely, most specifically in the hands.

Head: Thickset jaw, protruding brow line.

Eyes: Mildly diminished peripheral vision on visual fields by confrontation bilaterally; EOMs intact in six cardinal positions of gaze; PERRLA bilaterally.

ENT/Mouth: Slight gap between two front teeth; hypertrophy of pharyngeal soft tissues.

Neck: No abnormalities of thyroid on palpation.

Lungs: Clear to auscultation bilaterally.

Heart: No murmurs, gallops, or rub; RRR; PMI displaced laterally.

Genital/Rectal: Deferred.

Musculoskeletal: Prominence of bony structures in joints of hands, upper extremities, and lower extremities; widened joints and enlarged soft tissue structure around multiple joints; slight hyper-mobility in joints of upper and lower extremities as noted on ROS evaluation; crepitus present in bilateral knees on flexion and extension; hands and feet are enlarged (widened) compared proportionately to the height of the patient.

Neurologic: Sensation intact to light and sharp touch in upper and lower extremities; strength 5/5 in upper and lower extremities bilaterally; DTRs 2+ for tricep, bicep, brachioradialis, patellar, and Achilles reflexes bilaterally; negative Babinski sign; no increased or decreased tone on passive movement of limbs.

CLINICAL DISCUSSION QUESTIONS

1. What is the differential diagnosis?

_____

_____

_____

2. What is the most likely diagnosis? Why?

_____

_____

_____

_____

3. Demonstrate your understanding of the pathophysiology in regard to the most likely diagnosis.

_____

_____

_____

_____

4. Should tests/imaging studies be ordered? Which ones? Why? Think about tests/imaging beyond the primary care setting as well.

_____

_____

_____

_____

5. What are the next appropriate steps in management?

_____

_____

_____

_____

6. Review a recent and credible research article(s) about this diagnosis. Demonstrate your understanding of the underlying causes, associated conditions, and complications. Include a list of your reference(s).

_____

_____

_____

_____

7. What are the pertinent ICD-10 and CPT (E/M) codes for this visit? Provide a short rationale.

_____

_____

_____

_____

8. What is the appropriate patient education for this case?

_____

_____

_____

_____

9. If not managed appropriately, what is/are the medical/legal concern(s) that may arise?

_____

_____

_____

_____

10. Think about interprofessional collaboration for this case. Provide a list of specialties or other disciplines and indicate what contribution these professionals might make to managing the patient.

_____

_____

_____

_____

BEDSIDE MANNER QUESTIONS

11. What would your communication style/approach be with this patient?

_____

_____

_____

_____

12. If a patient is distressed by the diagnosis, what might offer support?

_____

_____

_____

_____

ANSWER KEY *available at*
https://connect.springerpub.com/content/book/978-0-8261-8273-9

FEVER AND LUMP ON NECK, ADOLESCENT MALE

CHIEF COMPLAINT

"Fever and lump on neck."

HISTORY OF PRESENT ILLNESS

A 13-year-old boy presents to an urban FQHC, reporting a lump on the left side of his neck, just below his ear, that has been there for 6 days. The patient speaks English, but his mother, who brings him to the clinic, speaks only Spanish. A trained medical Spanish interpreter attends the patient interview. The patient noticed a small bump on his neck one night 6 days ago, which became larger the following day. The next day a fever began. The fever was subjective, meaning the family did not take his temperature, but he felt feverish and was warm to the touch. On the evening of onset, he had a transient rash, which the mother describes as "hives." He complained of a sore throat the previous week but denies a sore throat currently. He does report slight dysphagia and mild headache.

He was seen 4 days earlier by another provider in the same clinic and started on amoxicillin for presumed bacterial lymphadenitis. At that time, he was febrile: 100.8°F (38.2°C). The mass is described as a 2.5- to 3-cm submandibular gland enlargement, which is firm and tender to palpation. A CBC was normal, and group A strep, mumps, and EBV testing were negative. Since that time, the patient thinks the lump has grown in size. His headache is somewhat improved, but he continues to be febrile.

REVIEW OF SYSTEMS

The patient's ROS is positive for a slight cough. His ROS is negative for abdominal pain, nausea, vomiting, or diarrhea. There is no eye discharge, pain, or irritation. There are no ear symptoms or nasal symptoms. There are no current skin symptoms, and the skin overlying the lump is not red or draining.

RELEVANT HISTORY

The patient's history is significant for atopic dermatitis, which has not been active within the past 6 months. There are no other known medical conditions. The patient has never been hospitalized, nor has ever had surgery. Immunizations are up to date.

The patient lives with his parents, who are married with two other children. The family is Spanish speaking, but the patient himself speaks fluent English. The family emigrated from El Salvador when the patient was a child. The patient is uninsured, and the family is on a sliding fee scale at the FQHC. The patient has two pet kittens who sleep in his bedroom. There are no other pets and no environmental tobacco smoke exposure. There has been no recent travel. The family lives in a home built within the past 30 years and has city water.

ALLERGIES

No known drug allergies. No known food allergies.

MEDICATIONS

- Amoxicillin 250 mg, PO TID for the past 4 days. Last dose was about 6 hours ago.
- Acetaminophen 325 mg, two tablets PO q8h. Last dose was about 6 hours ago.

PHYSICAL EXAMINATION

Vitals: T 37.2°C (99.0°F); P 77; R 16; BP 103/60; HT 157.5 cm (62 in.), 30th percentile; WT 45 kg. (99 lbs), 31st percentile; BMI 18.2, 38th percentile.

General: Alert and oriented, in no acute distress, with obvious swelling on the left jaw line at the angle of the mandible.

Psychiatric: Appropriate interaction for age. Affect is full and mood is regular.

Skin, Hair, Nails: Scattered superficial abrasions noted on bilateral upper extremities, which patient states are from his kittens and do not hurt. No abnormal findings with hair or nails.

Eyes: Sclerae clear.

ENT/Mouth: Ear canals are patent, and TMs are clear. Mouth mucosa is pink and moist without erythema, inflammation, or exudate.

Neck: Some limit to ROM secondary to a firm, but not hard, mobile 3×4-cm left-sided submandibular mass. The mass is tender to palpation without significant overlying induration or erythema but is slightly warm to the touch. There is no other anterior, occipital, or supraclavicular lymphadenopathy appreciated.

Lungs: Clear to auscultation bilaterally.

Heart: RRR without murmur, rubs, or gallops.

Abdomen: Soft, non-tender, non-distended, with no organomegaly.

Genital/Rectal: Deferred.

Neurologic: No focal deficits. Cranial nerves II to XII are normal.

CLINICAL DISCUSSION QUESTIONS

1. What is the differential diagnosis?

_____

_____

_____

_____

2. What is the most likely diagnosis? Why?

_____

_____

_____

_____

3. Demonstrate your understanding of the pathophysiology in regard to the most likely diagnosis.

_____

_____

_____

_____

4. Should tests/imaging studies be ordered? Which ones? Why? Think about tests/imaging beyond the primary care setting as well.

_____

_____

_____

_____

5. What are the next appropriate steps in management?

_____

_____

_____

_____

6. What is the treatment approach for this diagnosis? Provide references for your response.

_____

_____

_____

_____

7. What are the pertinent ICD-10 and CPT (E/M) codes for this visit? Provide a short rationale.

_____

_____

_____

_____

8. What are the appropriate patient/parent education topics for this case?

_____

_____

_____

_____

9. If not managed appropriately, what is/are the medical/legal concern(s) that may arise?

_____

_____

_____

_____

10. Think about interprofessional collaboration for this case. Provide a list of specialties or other disciplines and indicate what contribution these professionals might make to managing the patient.

_____

_____

_____

_____

BEDSIDE MANNER QUESTION

11. What would your communication style/approach be with this parent and patient?

_____

_____

_____

_____

ANSWER KEY _available at_
https://connect.springerpub.com/content/book/978-0-8261-8273-9

HAND PAIN AT NIGHT, ADULT FEMALE

CHIEF COMPLAINT

"Hand pain at night."

HISTORY OF PRESENT ILLNESS

A right-hand-dominant 64-year-old woman presents to her PCP for evaluation of right-hand pain. Her pain started 4 months ago and was initially noted as "just tingling" in the early morning hours while she was sleeping. At first, the symptoms did not radiate and remained localized to the base of her thumb and her index finger on the right hand. Over time, the patient noted an earlier onset of the paresthesia at night, and it began waking her several times per night. She attempted to sleep with her wrists extended because it was the only comfortable position. Inevitably, as she slept, her hand position would change, and her symptoms reoccurred. In the past few weeks, she has experienced a burning pain in her hand. It is affecting the thumb, index, and middle fingers of her right hand, with some radiation of symptoms to the wrist and lower forearm. She has noted decreased strength in the right hand, which is affecting her pastime of knitting. She stretches the wrist or "lets my hands hang to my side" to alleviate symptoms but the pain always returns. She denies any trauma or inciting event prior to the onset of symptoms. She has never experienced this type of pain/symptom in the past.

REVIEW OF SYSTEMS

The patient's ROS is positive for numbness/tingling in the median distribution of the right hand, weakness including dropping objects, or difficultly grasping cups or utensils for long periods. The ROS is negative for fatigue, weight loss, and night sweats. She denies neck pain or radiation of pain that originates from the cervical spine; she also denies joint pain in the elbow or shoulder of either upper extremity.

RELEVANT HISTORY

The patient's medical history is significant for HTN well controlled with lisinopril and type 2 diabetes mellitus (DM) well controlled with metformin. Her social history includes 2 glasses of red wine per week with friends at their card game. No history of tobacco use or illicit drug use now or in the past is reported. She is a retired elementary school teacher. Her family history includes mother, deceased, at age 78, CVA; father, deceased, at 82, complications from cancer. She has one twin sister, with HTN and type 2 DM as well, and three adult children all alive and well. She has been married to her husband for 42 years.

ALLERGIES

No known drug allergies; no known food allergies.

MEDICATIONS

- Lisinopril 10 mg PO QD.
- Metformin 500 mg PO BID.

PHYSICAL EXAMINATION

Vitals: T 37°C (98.6°F), P 62, R 16, BP 132/84, HT 162.56 cm (64 in.), WT 71.2 kg (157 lbs.), BMI 27.

General: Well-nourished, pleasant female with no acute distress.

Psychiatric: Cooperative on exam.

Skin, Hair, and Nails: Warm, dry, no apparent rashes. No abnormal findings with hair or nails.

Neck: Supple without tenderness to palpation or enlargement of thyroid.

Peripheral Vascular: Radial pulses intact; capillary refill brisk with no discoloration of the hand or fingers bilaterally.

Musculoskeletal: Positive Tinel sign in right wrist, negative in left; positive Phalen after 30 seconds of holding posture; ROM full in fingers, wrists, elbows, and shoulders bilaterally. Neck FROM with no elicitation of symptoms with flexion/extension/rotation of the cervical spine. Grip strength reduced 4/5 in the right hand and reduced compared to non-dominant left hand. Atrophy of the thenar eminence in the right hand in comparison to the left hand.

Neurologic: Diminished pinprick and light touch sensation in the right hand in the median nerve distribution; upper and lower extremity reflexes equal and symmetrical bilaterally (2+).

CLINICAL DISCUSSION QUESTIONS

1. What is the differential diagnosis?

_____

_____

_____

_____

2. What is the most likely diagnosis? Why?

_____

_____

_____

_____

3. Demonstrate your understanding about the pathophysiology in regard to the most likely diagnosis.

_____

_____

_____

_____

4. Should tests/imaging studies be ordered? Which ones? Why? Think about tests/imaging beyond the primary care setting as well.

_____

_____

_____

_____

5. What are the next appropriate steps in management?

_____

_____

_____

_____

6. What are the causes, comorbidities, incidence, and treatment options for this diagnosis? Provide references for your response.

_____

_____

_____

_____

7. What are the pertinent ICD-10 and CPT (E/M) codes for this visit? Provide a short rationale.

_____

_____

_____

_____

8. What is the appropriate patient education for this case?

_____

_____

_____

_____

9. If not managed appropriately, what is/are the medical/legal concern(s) that may arise?

_____

_____

_____

_____

10. Think about interprofessional collaboration for this case. Provide a list of specialties or other disciplines and indicate what contribution these professionals might make to managing the patient.

_____

_____

_____

_____

BEDSIDE MANNER QUESTIONS

11. What would your communication style/approach be with this patient?

_____

_____

_____

_____

12. If the patient is distressed by the diagnosis, what might offer support?

_____

_____

_____

_____

ANSWER KEY *available at*
https://connect.springerpub.com/content/book/978-0-8261-8273-9

BURNING WITH URINATION, ADULT MALE

CHIEF COMPLAINT

"Burning with urination."

HISTORY OF PRESENT ILLNESS

A 21-year-old man presents as a new patient for an evaluation of burning with urination for 3 days. He states he noticed it to be mild at first and thought maybe it was just irritation from a new soap he was using, but then it worsened. He also notes a small amount of clear penile discharge. When he had these same symptoms a few months ago, he went to a local DOH and was given antibiotics but does not remember the name. His symptoms went away immediately after treatment then, and he has been fine until this present concern. The patient's sexual history reveals he is active with both women and men but predominantly men. He has no current primary sexual partner, and he states having about five male sexual partners in the past 3 months. When he does have sex with men, he states he is primarily a "top" (insertive) partner with anal sex and both give and receive oral sex. Regarding condom use, he says he never uses condoms with oral sex and does not always use condoms during anal sex, depending on how much he trusts his partner. His last HIV test was 4 months ago during a student testing initiative; it was negative.

REVIEW OF SYSTEMS

Positive ROS findings as noted in the HPI. The ROS is negative for fever, chills, SOB, chest pain, abdominal pain, or rash.

RELEVANT HISTORY

The patient's medical history is significant for mild intermittent reactive airway disease controlled with an albuterol inhaler PRN. He uses an inhaler only occasionally, about once every couple of months. He is a social drinker at parties on weekends, rarely uses marijuana or edibles, and has no history of tobacco use or vaping. He has had no surgeries and is a senior in college with plans to pursue a PhD when he graduates. He denies any experimentation or use of other substances like methamphetamines, cocaine, opiates, or others. His family history is noncontributory.

ALLERGIES

No known drug allergies; no known food allergies.

MEDICATIONS

Albuterol inhaler 2 puffs every 4–6 hours PRN.

PHYSICAL EXAMINATION

Vitals: T 36°C (97°F), P 82, R 12, BP 113/82, WT 100.7 kg (222 lbs), H 180.3 cm (71 in.), BMI 31.
General: Thin male in no acute distress.
Psychiatric: Slightly anxious behavior noted.
Skin, Hair, and Nails: No notable rashes or lesions.
Abdomen: Soft, non tender, not distended, active bowel sounds, no masses felt.

Genital/Rectal: Uncircumcised male, able to retract foreskin easily. Clear discharge when instructed to milk the shaft. No lesions or rashes noted. Shotty bilateral inguinal lymphadenopathy noted, scrotum with mild tenderness when palpating left testicle. Both testicles are smooth with no evidence of masses or nodules. Valsalva maneuver reveals no hernia on either side. Rectal exam deferred.

CLINICAL DISCUSSION QUESTIONS

1. What is the differential diagnosis?

_____

_____

_____

_____

2. What is the most likely diagnosis? Why?

_____

_____

_____

_____

3. Demonstrate your understanding about the pathophysiology in regard to the most likely diagnosis.

_____

_____

_____

_____

4. Should tests/imaging studies be ordered? Which ones? Why? Think about tests/imaging beyond the primary care setting as well.

_____

_____

_____

_____

5. What are the next appropriate steps in management?

_____

_____

_____

_____

6. What are the testing recommendations, treatment options, and screening guidelines for this diagnosis? Provide references for your response.

_____

_____

_____

_____

7. What are the pertinent ICD-10 and CPT (E/M) codes for this visit? Provide a short rationale.

_____

_____

_____

_____

8. What is the appropriate patient education for this case?

_____

_____

_____

_____

9. If not managed appropriately, what is/are the medical/legal concern(s) that may arise?

_____

_____

_____

_____

10. Think about interprofessional collaboration for this case. Provide a list of specialties or other disciplines and indicate what contribution these professionals might make to managing the patient.

_____

_____

_____

_____

BEDSIDE MANNER QUESTIONS

11. What would your communication style/approach be with this patient?

_____

_____

_____

_____

12. If a patient is distressed by the diagnosis, what might offer support?

_____

_____

_____

_____

CONSTIPATION, ADULT FEMALE

CHIEF COMPLAINT

"Constipation."

HISTORY OF PRESENT ILLNESS

A 58-year-old woman with a complicated history of chronic low back pain, bipolar disorder, mixed anxiety, and depressive disorder presents to her PCP, a PA, complaining of constipation for several months. Constipation has been intermittent and has gotten worse over the past few weeks. She is now having a bowel movement about once every 4 days; her stools are hard and painful, and she has bright red blood on the toilet paper after she wipes. She does not feel she is able to completely evacuate her bowels. She denies melena, abdominal pain, bloating or excessive gas, loose stools, or fecal incontinence. She is afraid to take medications and has not tried any over-the-counter treatments for fear of side effects. She has had no changes in her regular medications and no short-acting narcotics for breakthrough pain. She reports a regular diet (lean protein, fruits/vegetables, grains) without changes; she admits to not drinking enough water, about 20 ounces daily; she denies caffeine or alcohol use. Her stress level has not increased; she admits to daily anxiety that limits her activities and reports anxiety is at baseline. She has never had a colonoscopy due to anxiety about the procedure and potential outcomes. Her chronic low back pain has been stable for the past 6 years with current medications; she has been on the same dose of extended-release morphine sulfate for 4 years. She fears discontinuing morphine sulfate will result in worsened back pain. She does not exercise, does not receive physical therapy, and is not followed by pain management.

REVIEW OF SYSTEMS

A ROS is positive for constipation, bright red blood per rectum, and anxiety. The ROS is negative for fever, night sweats, weight changes, fatigue; hair or skin changes, heat, or cold intolerance; and belching, halitosis, heartburn, early satiety, nausea, or vomiting. The patient was also negative for chest pain, palpitations, SOB, mania, ideas of grandiosity, hallucinations, suicidal ideations, and worsening anxiety or panic.

RELEVANT HISTORY

The patient's medical history is significant for asthma (since childhood), bipolar disorder (age 25), mixed anxiety and depressive disorder (age 45), GERD (age 50), hyperlipidemia (age 52), hypothyroidism secondary to lithium use (age 42; TSH last checked 3 months ago, in normal range), IBS-C, (age 48), chronic low back pain (age 52), psoriasis (age 23), diverticulitis (last episode 2 years ago, diet controlled), and primary hyperparathyroidism with hypercalcemia post partial resection 15 months ago (serum calcium level in normal range 3 months ago). Her social history includes no use of alcohol, tobacco, or recreational drugs. She is married with no children; she volunteers at her church, sings in the choir, and performs charity work with older people. Her family history is noncontributory.

ALLERGIES

Penicillin (hives); no known food allergies.

Medications

- Levothyroxine 75 mcg, PO QD.
- Omeprazole, extended release 40 mg PO QD.
- Morphine sulfate, extended release 60 mg PO QD.
- Lithium 300 mg, PO QD.
- Clonazepam 1 mg, PO qhs PRN insomnia/anxiety.
- Desonide 0.05% topical ointment, apply sparingly to affected area(s) BID.
- Albuterol inhaler, inhale two puffs q4h PRN, wheezing, dyspnea.

Physical Examination

Vitals: T 37°C (98.6°F), P 76, R 12, BP 115/74, HT 152 cm (60 in.), WT 62 kg (138 lbs), BMI 27.

General: Well-developed, well-nourished female in no apparent distress.

Psychiatric: Anxious, no pressured speech, good eye contact, good insight, no suicidal ideation.

Skin, Hair, and Nails: Mild psoriasis in ears, scalp; skin is warm and dry, no edema or rash; no hair or eyebrow thinning; no nail pits or splitting.

Neck: Well-healed scar from parathyroid surgery, normal thyroid/neck exam.

Lungs: Clear to auscultation bilaterally.

Heart: RRR, no murmurs, rubs, or gallops; no peripheral edema.

Abdomen: Soft, non-tender, non-distended, active bowel sounds in all quadrants, no hepatosplenomegaly or masses.

Musculoskeletal: Lumbosacral region without tenderness or muscle spasm, limited active range of motion in lumbar spine.

Neurologic: Lower extremity sensation intact, DTR 2+ patella, Achilles; negative SLR bilaterally.

Clinical Discussion Questions

1. What is the differential diagnosis?

_____

_____

_____

_____

2. What is the most likely diagnosis? Why?

_____

_____

_____

_____

3. Demonstrate your understanding about the pathophysiology in regard to the most likely diagnosis.

_____

_____

_____

_____

4. Should tests/imaging studies be ordered? Which ones? Why? Think about tests/imaging beyond the primary care setting as well.

_____

_____

_____

_____

5. What are the next appropriate steps in management?

_____

_____

_____

_____

6. What are the treatment options for this diagnosis? Provide references for your response.

_____

_____

_____

_____

7. What are the pertinent ICD-10 and CPT (E/M) codes for this visit? Provide a short rationale.

_____

_____

_____

_____

_____

8. What is the appropriate patient education topic for this case?

_____

_____

_____

_____

9. If not managed appropriately, what is/are the medical/legal concern(s) that may arise?

_____

_____

_____

_____

10. Think about interprofessional collaboration for this case. Provide a list of specialties or other disciplines and indicate what contribution these professionals might make to managing the patient.

_____

_____

_____

_____

BEDSIDE MANNER QUESTIONS

11. What would your communication style/approach be with this patient?

_____

_____

_____

_____

12. If a patient is distressed by the diagnosis, what might offer support?

_____

_____

_____

_____

ANSWER KEY _available at_
https://connect.springerpub.com/content/book/978-0-8261-8273-9

RECURRENT VOMITING, PEDIATRIC FEMALE

CHIEF COMPLAINT
"Recurrent vomiting."

HISTORY OF PRESENT ILLNESS

A mother presents with her 3-year-old daughter for an evaluation of recurrent vomiting. At the time of her first office visit, she had a 3- to 4-day history of one or two episodes of vomiting daily. There were no associated symptoms and she had no ill contacts. A physical examination of the skin, ears, throat, neck, thorax, and abdomen showed no abnormalities. A diagnosis of viral syndrome was made, and she was sent home with dietary modifications.

Despite slight improvement with dietary modifications, the child continued to have sporadic episodes of vomiting one to three times daily. She remained afebrile and apart from a decreased appetite had no new symptoms. Because of the persistent vomiting, she was seen in the clinic again 2 days later by a different provider. Her weight had decreased from 31 lbs to 29½ lbs, but she showed no signs of dehydration and her abdominal examination showed no abnormalities. At this visit, the provider discussed with the mother that although the time course of her vomiting was prolonged for a viral illness, she appeared well hydrated and had no concerning findings on abdominal examination. He mother was advised to encourage clear liquids and to offer small amounts of solids as tolerated. A follow-up appointment was scheduled for 3 days later.

The day before the scheduled follow-up appointment, the mother called the office concerned about the child's continued vomiting. The call was transferred to the provider who had seen her most recently, and her mother told the PCP, "I just know something is wrong. I'm afraid we're going to lose her." Because of this concern, the PCP recommended that the child be evaluated that same morning. Further history revealed that since her last visit, she had continued to have sporadic episodes of emesis, and when asked what concerned her most, her mother explained that this illness just seemed different from any she had experienced before. The vomiting seems to occur without warning, and she "just isn't acting herself."

REVIEW OF SYSTEMS

The patient's ROS is positive for weight loss, decreased appetite, and decreased activity. Her ROS is negative for fever, headache, nausea, abdominal pain, hematemesis, bilious emesis, cramping, diarrhea, or hematochezia.

RELEVANT HISTORY

The patient was diagnosed with GERD, diagnosed at age 6 months; she was treated with frequent, smaller feedings, and thickening formula. The GERD resolved by 15 months of age.

ALLERGIES

No known drug allergies; no known food allergies.

MEDICATIONS

None.

PHYSICAL EXAMINATION

Vitals: T 37°C (98.4°F), P 94, R 22, BP 90/50, HT 86 cm (34 in.), WT 12.7 kg (28 lbs), BMI 17.0.

General: Alert, sitting comfortably on mother's lap.

Skin, Hair, and Nails: No rash or skin lesions, normal skin turgor.

Eyes: No conjunctival injection or scleral icterus, pupils equal and reactive to light.

ENT/Mouth: Oropharynx without lesions, mucosa moist.

Neck: FROM, non-tender, no lymphadenopathy.

Lungs: Clear to auscultation bilaterally.

Heart: RRR, S1 and S2 normal intensity, no murmur or extra heart sounds.

Abdomen: Non-distended; normal quality and frequency of bowel sounds; soft, non-tender to deep palpation; no mass or hepatosplenomegaly.

Neurologic: Cranial nerves II to XII intact bilaterally, normal strength upper and lower extremity, gait wide based and unsteady.

CLINICAL DISCUSSION QUESTIONS

1. What is the differential diagnosis?

_____

_____

_____

_____

2. What is the most likely diagnosis? Why?

_____

_____

_____

_____

3. Demonstrate your understanding about the pathophysiology in regard to the most likely diagnosis.

_____

_____

_____

_____

4. Should tests/imaging studies be ordered? Which ones? Why? Think about tests/imaging beyond the primary care setting as well.

_____

_____

_____

_____

5. What are the next appropriate steps in management?

_____

_____

_____

_____

6. Review a credible research article/s on about this diagnosis. Demonstrate your understanding of the prevalence, treatment options, and risks. Provide your reference(s).

_____

_____

_____

_____

7. What are the pertinent ICD-10 and CPT (E/M) codes for this visit? Provide a short rationale.

_____

_____

_____

_____

8. What are the appropriate patient education topics for this case?

_____

_____

_____

_____

9. If not managed appropriately, what is/are the medical/legal concern(s) that may arise?

_____

_____

_____

_____

10. Think about interprofessional collaboration for this case. Provide a list of specialties or other disciplines and indicate what contribution these professionals might make to managing the patient.

_____

_____

_____

_____

BEDSIDE MANNER QUESTIONS

11. What would your communication style/approach be with this parent and child?

_____

_____

_____

_____

12. If a parent and child are distressed by the diagnosis, what might offer support?

_____

_____

_____

_____

ANSWER KEY _available at_
https://connect.springerpub.com/content/book/978-0-8261-8273-9

FATIGUE AND GENERAL MALAISE, ADULT MALE

CHIEF COMPLAINT

"Fatigue, general malaise."

HISTORY OF PRESENT ILLNESS

A 55-year-old man presents to his PCP with his wife after a 4-hour history of "feeling bad." This began suddenly while at home. He feels tired and does not want to do anything other than sit in his chair. He is winded quickly when he is moving around and feels like he has an upset stomach and believes it is indigestion. However, his wife notes he is not himself and she is worried about him. Upon further questioning, he does state he has pain and it is more over his chest than his abdomen. It does not radiate to his arm or neck. He has a hard time rating the pain, stating, "It just hurts." His best description of the pain is that it is dull. Sitting in his recliner seems to ease his pain. He is on hydrocodone/acetaminophen 10/325 mg for chronic lower-back pain, and this has not relieved his current symptoms. He has not wanted to eat anything today due to fatigue. His wife also notes he appears sweaty even though he has not done much all day.

The patient admits he has not been faithfully checking his blood pressure as he was asked to do on a prior visit. When he does check, which is approximately once a week, it is in the range of 140 to 150 for systolic; he does not know his diastolic blood pressure. His last cholesterol level was checked 4 months ago, and his LDL was mildly elevated at 140; total cholesterol, HDL and triglycerides were within normal limits.

REVIEW OF SYSTEMS

A ROS is positive for fatigue, loss of appetite, chest pain, SOB on exertion, anxiety, and chronic lower-back pain. The review is negative for fever, rhinorrhea, sore throat, ear pain, palpitations, edema of lower legs, orthopnea, wheezing, stridor, cough, nausea and vomiting, diarrhea, constipation, neck pain/stiffness, gait problems, depression, hallucinations, loss of consciousness, numbness, or weakness.

RELEVANT HISTORY

The patient's medical history includes hypercholesterolemia, hypertension, obesity, chronic lower-back pain, and generalized anxiety. He had a lumbar discectomy at age 44. He lives with his wife; they are happy. He is sexually active and in a monogamous relationship with his wife. He drinks a few beers over the weekend; he quit smoking 10 years ago but has a 1-pack-per-day history for 20 years. He admits to marijuana usage about a month ago. His father was diagnosed with CAD, at an unknown age; he is deceased.

ALLERGIES

No known drug allergies; no known food allergies.

MEDICATIONS

- Atorvastatin 10 mg PO QD.
- Hydrocodone/acetaminophen 10/325 mg PO QID PRN.
- Lisinopril 10 mg PO QD.
- Alprazolam 0.5 mg PO QID PRN.

PHYSICAL EXAMINATION

Vitals: T 37°C (98.6°F), P 94, R 16, BP 140/85, O2 95%, WT 117 kg (258 lbs), HT 177.8 cm (70 in.), BMI 37.

General: Appears sweaty and uncomfortable. Patient is obese.

Psychiatric: Anxious.

Skin, Hair, and Nails: Cool to touch and damp, pink, no pallor noted. No abnormal findings with hair or nails.

Lungs: Breathing is non-labored. He is not using accessory muscles for breathing, and there are no retractions noted. Lung fields are clear to auscultation bilaterally with good air movement; no wheezes, crackles, or rales noted.

Heart: RRR, no murmur or extra sounds noted. Chest is non-tender to palpation.

Vascular: Radial and pedal pulses are 2+ bilaterally. He has capillary refill time <2 seconds in fingers and toes. There is no edema noted in his extremities. No cyanosis is noted around mouth or in extremities. JVD is not noted.

Abdomen: BS normal. Soft, non-tender, no distension.

Neurologic: Cranial nerves II to XII grossly intact. Patient is A&O×3.

CLINICAL DISCUSSION QUESTIONS

1. What is the differential diagnosis?

_____

_____

_____

2. What is the most likely diagnosis? Why?

_____

_____

_____

3. Demonstrate your understanding about the pathophysiology in regard to the most likely diagnosis.

_____

_____

_____

4. Should tests/imaging studies be ordered? Which ones? Why? Think about tests/imaging beyond the primary care setting as well.

_____

_____

_____

_____

5. What are the next appropriate steps in management?

_____

_____

_____

_____

6. What are the risk predictors and symptom duration of the diagnosis? Provide references for your response.

_____

_____

_____

_____

7. What are the pertinent ICD-10 and CPT (E/M) codes for this visit? Provide a short rationale.

_____

_____

_____

_____

8. What is the appropriate patient education for this case?

_____

_____

_____

_____

9. If not managed appropriately, what is/are the medical/legal concern(s) that may arise?

_____

_____

_____

_____

10. Think about interprofessional collaboration for this case. Provide a list of specialties or other disciplines and indicate what contribution these professionals might make to managing the patient.

_____

_____

_____

_____

BEDSIDE MANNER QUESTIONS

11. What would your communication style/approach be with this patient and his wife?

_____

_____

_____

_____

12. If a patient and his wife are distressed by a diagnosis, what might offer support?

_____

_____

_____

_____

ANSWER KEY *available at*
https://connect.springerpub.com/content/book/978-0-8261-8273-9

NAUSEA, VOMITING, AND HEADACHE, ADOLESCENT MALE

CHIEF COMPLAINT

"Nausea, vomiting, and headache."

HISTORY OF PRESENT ILLNESS

A mother brings her 13-year-old son to his PCP for evaluation. He has a 1-day history of nausea, vomiting, and headache with photosensitivity. He is in the 8th grade, doing well in school, and active in community sports. In a football game yesterday, the front of his head connected with another player's shoulder pads; his head whipped back, he lost his balance, and he fell to the ground hitting the back of his head. His mother helps recount the accident, as the patient does not remember all the details. No loss of consciousness was noted. After a brief rest on the sidelines, he continued minimal play. The team went for pizza after the game; during dinner he complained of a headache. Upon arriving at home, he had two to three episodes of nausea/vomiting. The headache continued with photosensitivity. Today, he has continued nausea, with no further vomiting; headache is still present, and he states, "My balance is a bit off."

REVIEW OF SYSTEMS

The patient's ROS is positive for nausea, vomiting, headache, mild visual changes, and mild balance disturbances. His ROS is negative for sleep difficulty or excessive sleep, difficulty concentrating, irritability, or sadness, numbness, or tingling.

RELEVANT HISTORY

The boy was born via Cesarean section at term, 8 lbs, 19.5 in., history of newborn GERD, which has resolved. He was the parents' first child. He lives with parents and siblings in a single-family home, with no family history of smoking. His family medical history is negative, except for the mom with thyroid removal surgery in 2010 for a nodular noncancerous thyroid.

ALLERGIES

No known drug allergies; no known food allergies.

MEDICATIONS

None.

PHYSICAL EXAMINATION

Vitals: T 37°C (98.7°F), P 98, BP 102/54, WT 59.3 kg (130.8 lbs), HT 157.5 cm (62 in.), BMI 23.9.

General: Alert and active in mild acute distress. Appears fatigued.

Psychiatric: Affect is normal and appropriate.

Head: Head is normocephalic.

Eyes: PERRL, red reflex present bilaterally, EOM full, positive nystagmus.

ENT/Mouth: Tympanic membranes pearly gray with visible cone of light and landmarks. Mucosa is pink and moist. Normal speech and tone. Uvula midline.

Lungs: Respirations even and unlabored, clear bilaterally.

Heart: Normal S1 S2 without rubs, murmurs, or gallops.

Musculoskeletal: Motor 5/5 proximal and distal upper and lower extremities, including shoulders. DTRs 2+ and symmetrical of knees, Achilles, brachioradialis, and biceps tendons. Gait normal, balance distorted with standing on one foot and heal toe walking, has pronator drift.

Neurologic: Cranial nerves II to XII grossly intact. Sensory grossly intact to light touch symmetrically.

CLINICAL DISCUSSION QUESTIONS

1. What is the differential diagnosis?

_____

_____

_____

_____

2. What is the most likely diagnosis? Why?

_____

_____

_____

_____

3. Demonstrate your understanding about the pathophysiology in regard to the most likely diagnosis.

_____

_____

_____

_____

4. Should tests/imaging studies be ordered? Which ones? Why? Think about tests/imaging beyond the primary care setting as well.

_____

_____

_____

_____

5. What are the next appropriate steps in management?

_____

_____

_____

_____

6. What are the prevalence, complications, and current guidelines post diagnosis? Provide references for your response.

_____

_____

_____

_____

7. What are the pertinent ICD-10 and CPT (E/M) codes for this visit? Provide a short rationale.

_____

_____

_____

_____

8. What is the appropriate patient education for this case?

_____

_____

_____

_____

9. If not managed appropriately, what is/are the medical/legal concern(s) that may arise?

_____

_____

_____

_____

10. Think about interprofessional collaboration for this case. Provide a list of specialties or other disciplines and indicate what contribution these professionals might make to managing the patient.

_____

_____

_____

_____

BEDSIDE MANNER QUESTIONS

11. What would your communication style/approach be with this patient and his mother?

_____

_____

_____

_____

12. If the patient and his mother are distressed by the diagnosis, what might offer support?

_____

_____

_____

_____

ANSWER KEY _available at_
https://connect.springerpub.com/content/book/978-0-8261-8273-9

DIZZINESS AND DIFFICULTY HEARING, ADULT MALE

CHIEF COMPLAINT
"Dizziness and hearing difficulty."

HISTORY OF PRESENT ILLNESS
A 64-year-old man presents to his PCP complaining of intermittent episodes of dizziness occurring over the past year. The dizziness, described as a spinning sensation, comes every 1 to 2 weeks and generally lasts for 6 to 12 hours. These episodes often are accompanied by nausea and vomiting. He has more recently noticed hearing fluctuations, especially in his left ear. The hearing loss is worse just before and during attacks and then improves. He also now describes a sense of aural fullness and tinnitus, described as a low-frequency blowing or roaring sound in the ear, associated with the episodes. He attributes these symptoms to noise exposure with his work. He has taken over-the-counter meclizine to help with the dizziness, with some relief of the symptoms.

REVIEW OF SYSTEMS
The patient's ROS is positive for vertigo, tinnitus, hearing loss, nausea, and vomiting. He has occasional headaches that respond to treatment with acetaminophen. His ROS is negative for fever, chills, weight loss, or fatigue.

RELEVANT HISTORY
The patient has had no major illnesses, injuries, surgeries, or hospitalizations. He is a lifelong non-smoker and drinks one to two glasses of wine per week. He is employed as a high school music teacher and plays in a band part-time on weekends. The patient is married and has three grown children who are all in good health. His family history is significant for hypertension in both parents. There is no family history of cancer, early heart disease, or diabetes.

ALLERGIES
No known medical allergies; no known drug allergies.

MEDICATIONS
- Meclizine 25 mg PO TID OTC, PRN.
- Acetaminophen, 500 mg PRN.

PHYSICAL EXAMINATION
Vitals: T 37°C (98.6°F), P 76, R 14, BP 132/82, HT 177.8 cm (70 in.), WT 81.65 kg (180 lbs), BMI 25.8.

General: Well-developed and nourished 64-year-old male patient in no acute distress.

Psychiatric: Appears mildly anxious.

Skin, Hair, and Nails: Skin warm and dry, no rashes or bleeding tendency. No abnormal findings with hair or nails.

ENT/Mouth: TMs appear pearly, gray with no fluid noted. Hearing is decreased in the left ear as compared to the right on gross testing. Oral mucosa is moist; dentition in good repair with no caries or erosions.

Neck: Supple with no adenopathy or thyroid enlargement.

Lungs: Clear to auscultation bilaterally.

Heart: RRR, without murmur, gallop, or rub.

Abdomen: Soft with no masses, organomegaly, or tenderness. Active bowel sounds heard in all quadrants.

Neurologic: A&O×3; immediate, recent, and remote memory intact; Cranial nerves II–XII grossly intact; strength 3/5 and DTRs 2+ symmetrical in all extremities; sensation, coordination, balance, cerebellar function, and gait intact.

CLINICAL DISCUSSION QUESTIONS

1. What is the differential diagnosis?

_____

_____

_____

_____

2. What is the most likely diagnosis? Why?

_____

_____

_____

_____

3. Demonstrate your understanding about the pathophysiology in regard to the most likely diagnosis.

_____

_____

_____

_____

4. Should tests/imaging studies be ordered? Which ones? Why? Think about tests/imaging beyond the primary care setting as well.

_____

_____

_____

_____

5. What are the next appropriate steps in management?

_____

_____

_____

_____

6. What are the diagnostic criteria and treatment options for this diagnosis? Provide references for your response.

_____

_____

_____

_____

_____

7. What are the pertinent ICD-10 and CPT (E/M) codes for this visit? Provide a short rationale.

_____

_____

_____

_____

_____

8. What is the appropriate patient education for this case?

_____

_____

_____

_____

_____

9. If not managed appropriately, what is/are the medical/legal concern(s) that may arise?

_____

_____

_____

_____

_____

10. Think about interprofessional collaboration for this case. Provide a list of specialties or other disciplines and indicate what contribution these professionals might make to managing the patient.

_____

_____

_____

_____

_____

BEDSIDE MANNER QUESTION

11. What would be your communication style/approach with this patient?

_____

_____

_____

_____

_____

ANSWER KEY _available at_
https://connect.springerpub.com/content/book/978-0-8261-8273-9

BAD HEADACHE, ADULT FEMALE

CHIEF COMPLAINT

"Bad headache."

HISTORY OF PRESENT ILLNESS

A 48-year-old woman presents to her PCP with a 2-day history of a bad headache. She asks the lights to be turned off in the exam room to lessen the pain. Her pain began yesterday morning an hour after awakening. She reports seeing "zigzags of lights" in her vision for several minutes before the headache pain began and grew over 2 hours, rated them as 8/10, now rated 5/10. She points to her left temple and states it is an "intense, steady pain." She reports nausea with two episodes of vomiting yesterday, with a more throbbing pain that made it difficult to sleep. Taking 1,000 mg acetaminophen helps, but any relief only lasts a couple of hours. She has had this type of headache before (including the visual disturbance) but it never lasted this long. Her last headache was about a month ago, lasting less than a day. The patient is a graduate student in her third of five semesters, lives with an older sister, and works as a barista evenings and weekends. She cannot work or study with this headache. She is on oral birth control but on no other medications and admits to increased stress due to finances, a fight with her boyfriend, and intense studies.

REVIEW OF SYSTEMS

The patient's ROS is positive for headache, nausea/vomiting, and visual changes. Significant negatives are an absence of fever, congestion, dizziness, or extremity weakness.

RELEVANT HISTORY

The patient is "generally healthy" and denies recent illness. By clinic record, her only surgery was a laparoscopic appendectomy at age 13 with no complications. She reports two to three beers/week and smokes marijuana one to two times a month. Her parents are divorced; her mother has type 2 diabetes and her father has hypertension and prostate cancer (under treatment). Her mother has always had similar headaches, saying, "There's nothing that can be done but to wait it out." There is no family history of cranial bleeding or other cancers.

ALLERGIES

No known medical allergies; no known food allergies.

MEDICATIONS

1,000 mg acetaminophen PRN.

PHYSICAL EXAMINATION

Vitals: T 37°C (98.6°F), P 84, R 18, BP 110/70, HT 157.5 cm (62 in.), WT 60.8 kg (134 lbs), BMI 24.5.

General: Moderate distress consistent with chief complaint, well-nourished, cooperative adult.

Psychiatric: Appropriate concern for health.

Skin, Hair, and Nails: No rashes or lesions. No abnormal findings with hair or nails.

Eyes: PERRLA, visual fields full, fundi negative for hemorrhages, disc margins sharp.

Lungs: Clear to auscultation bilaterally.

Heart: RRR without murmur.

Abdomen: Soft without tenderness, no hepatomegaly, spleen/kidneys not palpable.

Neurologic: A&O×3, CN II–XII grossly intact, Romberg negative, extremity DTRs 2+/4+, muscle strength symmetrically equal in extremities.

CLINICAL DISCUSSION QUESTIONS

1. What is the differential diagnosis?

_____

_____

_____

_____

2. What is the most likely diagnosis? Why?

_____

_____

_____

3. Demonstrate your understanding about the pathophysiology in regard to the most likely diagnosis.

_____

_____

_____

4. Should tests/imaging studies be ordered? Which ones? Why? Think about tests/imaging beyond the primary care setting as well.

_____

_____

_____

_____

5. What are the next appropriate steps in management?

_____

_____

_____

_____

6. What are the diagnostic criteria and treatment options for this diagnosis? Provide references for your response.

_____

_____

_____

7. What are the pertinent ICD-10 and CPT (E/M) codes for this visit? Provide a short rationale.

_____

_____

_____

_____

8. What is the appropriate patient education for this case?

_____

_____

_____

_____

9. If not managed appropriately, what is/are the medical/legal concern(s) that may arise?

_____

_____

_____

_____

10. Think about interprofessional collaboration for this case. Provide a list of specialties or other disciplines and indicate what contribution these professionals might make to managing the patient.

_____

_____

_____

_____

BEDSIDE MANNER QUESTION

11. What would be your communication style/approach with this patient?

_____

_____

_____

_____

ANSWER KEY *available at*
https://connect.springerpub.com/content/book/978-0-8261-8273-9

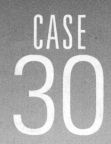

ABDOMINAL PAIN, ADULT FEMALE

CHIEF COMPLAINT
"Abdominal pain."

HISTORY OF PRESENT ILLNESS
A 53-year-old woman presents with complaints of gnawing and constant 6/10 abdominal pain that started the day prior. She states she is afraid to eat anything for fear the pain will worsen. She reports an episode similar to this occurring 5 years ago after returning home from overseas travel. She recalls being told by a physician that she probably had food poisoning, being given an antibiotic, and feeling better 2 to 3 days later. She says this has not happened since. She cannot think of anything she may have eaten that could have caused this pain, as it "came out of nowhere." Her last meal was a breakfast of rye toast and yogurt with blackberries yesterday.

She reports being very feverish, sweaty, and nauseated when the pain first started. She denies vomiting but does admit to a few of bouts of dry heaves. She is unable to point to where it hurts the most, stating, "It's all over." She admits to feeling bloated and having multiple bowel movements, with her last one just prior to presentation. She states her stools have gone from soft to loose thin ribbons and now nothing at all. She feels a need to evacuate her bowels but nothing comes out. She worries about having bloody stools similar to 5 years ago but has not seen that yet. She denies dysuria. She admits to having a high-stress job but denies ever being diagnosed with IBS or IBD. She has not traveled recently, nor has she been around anyone with similar symptoms. Her last colonoscopy was 5 years ago and was unremarkable.

REVIEW OF SYSTEMS
The patient's ROS is positive for subjective fever with chills, diaphoresis, difficulty sleeping due to abdominal pain, dry mouth, GERD, and reduced appetite. She denies recent unintentional weight loss or gain. Her ROS is negative for trouble swallowing, rectal bleeding, black or tarry stools, excessive belching or passing gas, liver problems, hepatitis, and jaundice.

RELEVANT HISTORY
The patient has a history of GERD, biliary dyskinesia with resultant laparoscopic cholecystectomy, uterine fibroids with resultant total abdominal hysterectomy, nephrolithiasis, and menopause. She drinks one to two glasses of wine with dinner two to three nights a week. Her family history is non-contributory.

ALLERGIES
Erythromycin results in hives; no known food allergies.

MEDICATIONS
- Pantoprazole 40 mg, PO QD.
- Calcium 600 mg PO BID.
- Vitamin D 800 IU PO BID.

PHYSICAL EXAMINATION

Vitals: T 37.7°C (99.8°F), P 86, R 14, BP 146/94, HT 173 cm (68 in.), WT 76 kg (168 lbs), BMI 25.5.

General: Well-dressed and well-nourished female who appears younger than stated age, in obvious discomfort laying in the fetal position on the examination table. She is alert and oriented.

Eyes: Non-icteric, sclera injected, conjunctiva pink bilaterally. PERRLA.

ENT/Mouth: Dry mucosa, no lesions, patent oropharynx, 1+ bilateral tonsils pink without exudate, uvula midline.

Neck: Supple, anterior cervical lymphadenopathy bilaterally.

Lungs: Clear to auscultation bilaterally.

Heart: +S1/S2, RRR, without murmurs, rubs, or gallops.

Peripheral Vascular: Warm throughout, all pulses 2+ symmetric bilaterally, capillary refill time < 2 seconds throughout.

Abdomen: Distended abdomen; well-healed surgical scars in the mid-epigastric region, RUQ, and suprapubic region. Hyperactive BS ×4; diffusely tender mid to LLQ with rebound tenderness; no thrills, no bruits, no costovertebral angle tenderness.

Genital/Rectal: (+) rectal tone, (+) guaiac, no external hemorrhoids.

Neurologic: Cranial nerves II to XII grossly intact, speech and gait appropriate.

CLINICAL DISCUSSION QUESTIONS

1. What is the differential diagnosis?

_____

_____

_____

_____

2. What is the most likely diagnosis? Why?

_____

_____

_____

_____

3. Demonstrate your understanding about the pathophysiology in regard to the most likely diagnosis.

_____

_____

_____

_____

4. Should tests/imaging studies be ordered? Which ones? Why? Think about tests/imaging beyond the primary care setting as well.

_____

_____

_____

_____

5. What are the next appropriate steps in management?

_____

_____

_____

_____

6. Review a reliable, recent reference regarding risk factors and treatment approaches for this diagnosis. Provide references for your response.

_____

_____

_____

_____

7. What are the pertinent ICD-10 and CPT (E/M) codes for this visit? Provide a short rationale.

_____

_____

_____

_____

8. What are appropriate patient education topics for this case?

_____

_____

_____

_____

9. If not managed appropriately, what is/are the medical/legal concern(s) that may arise?

_____

_____

_____

_____

10. Think about interprofessional collaboration for this case. Provide a list of specialties or other disciplines and indicate what contribution these professionals might make to managing the patient.

_____

_____

_____

_____

BEDSIDE MANNER QUESTION

11. What would your communication style/approach be with this patient?

_____

_____

_____

_____

ANSWER KEY *available at*
https://connect.springerpub.com/content/book/978-0-8261-8273-9

PAINFUL URINATION, ADULT MALE

CHIEF COMPLAINT

"Painful urination."

HISTORY OF PRESENT ILLNESS

A 32-year-old single man presents to his PCP with complaints of dysuria for the past week. He reports 8/10 burning with a painfully heavy sensation in his bladder and rectum, and he is unable to void except small amounts with great frequency throughout the day. He also complains of nocturia, which he denies ever occurred before. He reports a fever of 100.7°F (38.2°C) with chills that started yesterday. He admits to discomfort with bowel movements and is trying hard not to strain as the pain intensifies. He discloses having multiple female sexual partners and seldom uses condoms but relies on his partners to provide birth control. He was last sexually active 4 to 5 days ago, engaging in unprotected anal intercourse. He denies ever having STIs, blood in his urine, ejaculate or stool, penile discharge or pain, abdominal pain, and scrotal or testicular pain. He has not tried any over-the-counter medications to relieve his pain or fever.

REVIEW OF SYSTEMS

The patient's ROS is positive for increased frequency of urination with burning pain/pressure, nocturia, urgency, reduced caliber of stream, and hesitancy. He admits to fever, chills, malaise, and insomnia. His ROS is negative for nausea, vomiting, abdominal pain, change or frequency in bowel habits, rectal bleeding, hemorrhoids, constipation, diarrhea, or hepatitis. He denies kidney stones, hernias, penile discharge, lesions, testicular pain, masses, STIs, and exposure to HIV.

RELEVANT HISTORY

The patient has a history of hypercholesterolemia. He has smoked a pack of cigarettes a day for 10 years. He consumes 3 to 4 alcoholic drinks on the weekends. He denies any recreational or illicit drug use.

ALLERGIES

No known drug allergies; no known food allergies.

MEDICATIONS

Atorvastatin 20 mg PO QD.

PHYSICAL EXAMINATION

Vitals: T 38.4°C (101.2°F), P 104, R 14, BP 148/92, HT 188 cm (74 in.), WT 100.2 kg (221 lbs), BMI 28.4.

General: Well-developed, well-nourished male appearing of stated age laying in obvious discomfort on the examination table. He is alert and oriented, makes good eye contact and answers all questions appropriately.

Skin, Hair, and Nails: Consistently warm throughout, diaphoretic, without rashes, lesions, or masses.

ENT/Mouth: Good repair of teeth and gums, no bleeding. Dry mucosa without lesions or masses, patent oropharynx, uvula midline.

Neck: FROM, supple, anterior cervical and tonsillar adenopathy bilaterally.

Lungs: Clear to auscultation bilaterally, without wheezes.

Heart: +S1/S2, RRR, without murmurs, rubs, or gallops.

Abdomen: Protuberant, soft, BS ×4, tender at suprapubic aspect. Negative CVA tenderness.

Genital/Rectal: Circumcised male without urethral discharge, no scrotal masses, lesions or varicosities. (++) perineal pain, prostate firm, unable to determine the size (performed gently), hot to the touch, no masses, guaiac (−).

Musculoskeletal: FROM throughout without pain.

Neurologic: Cranial nerves II to XII grossly intact.

CLINICAL DISCUSSION QUESTIONS

1. What is the differential diagnosis?

_____

_____

_____

_____

2. What is the most likely diagnosis? Why?

_____

_____

_____

_____

3. Demonstrate your understanding about the pathophysiology in regard to the most likely diagnosis.

_____

_____

_____

_____

4. Should tests/imaging studies be ordered? Which ones? Why? Think about tests/imaging beyond the primary care setting as well.

_____

_____

_____

_____

5. What are the next appropriate steps in management?

_____

_____

_____

_____

6. What are the prevalence, risk factors, typical presentation, and complications of this diagnosis? Provide references for your response.

_____

_____

_____

_____

7. What are the pertinent ICD-10 and CPT (E/M) codes for this visit? Provide a short rationale.

_____

_____

_____

_____

8. What is the appropriate patient education for this case?

_____

_____

_____

_____

9. If not managed appropriately, what is/are the medical/legal concern(s) that may arise?

_____

_____

_____

_____

10. Think about interprofessional collaboration for this case. Provide a list of specialties or other disciplines and indicate what contribution these professionals might make to managing the patient.

_____

_____

_____

_____

BEDSIDE MANNER QUESTION
11. What would your communication style/approach be with this patient?

_____

_____

_____

_____

ANSWER KEY _available at_
https://connect.springerpub.com/content/book/978-0-8261-8273-9

7. ...

2. What are the normal ranges of and ... Provide a short rationale.

8. Why are ...

9. ...

10. Based ... diseases or conditions for which ...

11. ...

FREQUENT DIARRHEA, ADOLESCENT FEMALE

CHIEF COMPLAINT

"Frequent diarrhea."

HISTORY OF PRESENT ILLNESS

A 16-year-old young woman presents to her family PCP with her mother. The patient began having gastrointestinal symptoms 2 years ago following a camping trip with her family. At that time, both the patient and an older brother developed acute nausea, vomiting, abdominal pain, and diarrhea. No other family members were affected. The parents thought the children had a virus or food poisoning and treated them conservatively with oral fluid replacement and acetaminophen for low-grade fever. The brother's symptoms resolved quickly over the next 2 to 3 days; the patient's symptoms slowly improved in 1 week. However, since then, she has had recurrent episodes of lower abdominal cramping and pain, combined with loose to watery, non-bloody stools. At times she will have a sense of fecal urgency and tenesmus associated with the diarrhea. She also frequently feels bloated. Her symptoms have occurred at least 1 day per week for the past 6 months. The patient also has occasional headaches that respond well to treatment with acetaminophen. Her appetite and weight have remained stable, and no other symptoms have developed.

The family's PCP first saw her a few weeks after the initial illness because of recurring symptoms and has been seen in follow-up 2 to 3 times over the past year. During this time, several studies have been done: stool studies (ova and parasites, fecal leukocytes, routine stool cultures, and tests for *Giardia lamblia*), which were normal, and blood work (CBC, CMP, and CRP), which was normal. When her symptoms persisted, tests for celiac disease (serum TTG or tissue transglutaminase antibody and serum IgA) were done and were negative. The mother states they have avoided gluten and dairy products without long-term improvement. The only medication used is loperamide PRN. The use of loperamide has resulted in some improvement in the diarrhea, but the bloating and lower abdominal pain and cramps persist.

REVIEW OF SYSTEMS

A ROS was positive for the symptoms related in the HPI: abdominal pain, bloating, and diarrhea. The ROS was negative for fever, chills, vomiting, weight loss, urinary symptoms, and fatigue.

RELEVANT HISTORY

The patient has had no major illnesses, injuries, surgeries, or hospitalizations. Menstrual history: menarche at age 12. First day of LMP 14 days ago. Menses are regular, occurring every 28 to 30 days. Flow is moderate, lasting 5 to 7 days. She denies dysmenorrhea. She is not sexually active. There is no family history of cancer or IBD.

ALLERGIES

No known drug allergies; no known food allergies.

MEDICATIONS

Acetaminophen 500 mg PRN for fever and headaches.

PHYSICAL EXAMINATION

Vitals: T 37°C (98.6°F), P 76, R 14, BP 114/72, HT 165 cm (65 in.), WT 53.5 kg (118 lbs), BMI 19.6.

General: Well-developed and nourished 16-year-old female patient in no acute distress.

Psychiatric: Appears mildly anxious.

Skin, Hair, and Nails: Skin warm and dry, no rashes or bleeding tendency.

ENT/Mouth: Ears: TMs appear pearly; gray with no fluid noted. Oral mucosa is moist and dentition is in good repair with no caries or erosions.

Neck: Supple with no adenopathy or thyroid enlargement.

Lungs: Clear to auscultation bilaterally.

Heart: RRR, without murmur, gallop, or rub.

Abdomen: Soft with no masses, organomegaly, or tenderness. Active bowel sounds heard in all quadrants.

Genital/Rectal: Deferred.

Lymphatics: No axillary or inguinal lymphadenopathy.

Neurologic: A&O×3, cranial merves II to XII grossly intact.

CLINICAL DISCUSSION QUESTIONS

1. What is the differential diagnosis?

_____

_____

_____

_____

2. What is the most likely diagnosis? Why?

_____

_____

_____

_____

3. Demonstrate your understanding about the pathophysiology in regard to the most likely diagnosis.

_____

_____

_____

_____

4. Should tests/imaging studies be ordered? Which ones? Why? Think about tests/imaging beyond the primary care setting as well.

_____

_____

_____

_____

5. What are the next appropriate steps in management?

_____

_____

_____

_____

6. What are the diagnostic criteria and underlying conditions associated with the diagnosis? Include the name of the references.

_____

_____

_____

_____

7. What are the pertinent ICD-10 and CPT (E/M) codes for this visit? Provide a short rationale.

_____

_____

_____

_____

8. What are the appropriate patient education topics for this case?

_____

_____

_____

_____

9. If not managed appropriately, what is/are the medical/legal concern(s) that may arise?

_____

_____

_____

_____

10. Think about interprofessional collaboration for this case. Provide a list of specialties or other disciplines and indicate what contribution these professionals might make to managing the patient.

_____

_____

_____

_____

BEDSIDE MANNER QUESTIONS

11. What would your communication style/approach be with this patient and her mother?

_____

_____

_____

_____

12. If a patient and her mother are distressed by the diagnosis, what might offer support?

_____

_____

_____

_____

ANSWER KEY _available at_
https://connect.springerpub.com/content/book/978-0-8261-8273-9

REPETITIVE BRUISING ON LEGS, PEDIATRIC FEMALE

CHIEF COMPLAINT

"Repetitive bruising on legs."

HISTORY OF PRESENT ILLNESS

A mother and her 16-month-old daughter present to their pediatric office with a 2-week history of bruising. The mother says she started noticing bruises of different sizes mainly on the child's legs and thighs 2 weeks ago. After some bruises disappeared, new ones appeared. They start as purple spots and then change to brown before shrinking and disappearing. The child is walking now and stumbles, but no more so than any toddler. She is active and energetic without any recent trauma/accidents. She has been seen regularly in the clinic for all her routine well-child checks, and bruising was not noted at the last 15-month well-child check, when she received immunizations. The mother mentions that the child had a cold about 3 weeks ago, but the low-grade fever and sniffles resolved in a few days. Currently, her daughter has no other symptoms. She demonstrates normal growth, normal development, and a healthy diet.

REVIEW OF SYSTEMS

The child's ROS is positive for bruises on both lower extremities, recent viral illness 3 weeks ago, and routine vaccines 1 month ago. Her ROS is negative for fever, fatigue, nosebleeds, gingival bleeding, hematuria, hematochezia, change in appetite, energy, voids, stools, and new medications.

RELEVANT HISTORY

The child has no previously recorded or active medical problems. She lives at home with her parents and older sibling and attends day care 3 days a week. Family history is negative for cancer, bleeding disorders, and autoimmune disorders.

ALLERGIES

No known drug allergies; no known food allergies.

MEDICATIONS

None.

PHYSICAL EXAMINATION

Vitals: T 36.9°C (98.4°F); P 116; R 26; BP 100/60; WT 10.6 kg (23 lbs, 6 oz.), 75th percentile; HT 80 cm (31.5 in.), 75th percentile; HC 46.2 cm (18.1 in.).

General: Well appearing, interactive and playful, walking around the exam room, non-concerning interaction between parent and child.

Skin, Hair, and Nails: No excessive pallor, 10 to 12 purple–brown macules with irregular borders of varying sizes from 0.5 to 2 cm in diameter on bilateral legs and thighs, non-tender, non-blanching; also with 5 to 6 non-blanching, pinpoint, brightly erythematous macules on forehead and left cheek.

ENT/Mouth: Normal nasal turbinates with pink mucosa, no evidence of bleeding. Moist mucous membranes with no evidence of gingival bleeding, no thrush, normal pharynx.

Neck: No cervical lymphadenopathy.

Axilla: No axillary lymphadenopathy.

Abdomen: Soft, non-tender, non-distended, no hepatomegaly, no splenomegaly, no inguinal lymphadenopathy.

CLINICAL DISCUSSION QUESTIONS

1. What is the differential diagnosis?

_____

_____

_____

_____

2. What is the most likely diagnosis? Why?

_____

_____

_____

3. Demonstrate your understanding of the pathophysiology in regard to the most likely diagnosis.

_____

_____

_____

_____

4. Should tests/imaging studies be ordered? Which ones? Why? Think about tests/imaging beyond the primary care setting as well.

_____

_____

_____

_____

5. What are the next appropriate steps in management?

_____

_____

_____

6. What are the causes and prognosis of the diagnosis? Provide references for your responses.

_____

_____

_____

_____

7. What are the pertinent ICD-10 and CPT (E/M) codes for this visit? Provide a short rationale.

_____

_____

_____

_____

8. What are appropriate parent education topics for this case?

_____

_____

_____

_____

9. If not managed appropriately, what is/are the medical/legal concern(s) that may arise?

_____

_____

_____

_____

10. Think about interprofessional collaboration for this case. Provide a list of specialties or other disciplines and indicate what contribution these professionals might make to managing the patient.

_____

_____

_____

_____

Bedside Manner Questions

11. What would your communication style/approach be with this parent?

_____

_____

_____

_____

12. If a patient's mother is distressed by the diagnosis, what might offer support?

_____

_____

_____

_____

Answer Key _available at_
https://connect.springerpub.com/content/book/978-0-8261-8273-9

SWOLLEN KNEE, PEDIATRIC FEMALE

CHIEF COMPLAINT
"Swollen knee."

HISTORY OF PRESENT ILLNESS
An 11-year-old girl presents to her pediatrics office with her father complaining of left knee pain with warmth and swelling as well as a rash on her chest and both arms and legs for the past 2 days. She denies any known injury and denies joint locking or instability. She admits to generalized achiness and fatigue over the past week and a fever of 102.5F last night but denies chills or night sweats. She was seen by another provider in the practice 6 days prior for a sore throat and low-grade fever. Her sister had been diagnosed with group A strep on a rapid strep test, so amoxicillin 250 mg PO TID was prescribed without lab testing. The rash is not pruritic but is intermittent, occurring more at night when she has a fever. She denies changes in diet, soaps, or detergents. She takes no medications other than the current amoxicillin; she has taken amoxicillin previously without rash or reaction. She is generally well. She is a ballet dancer and has been on a heavy rehearsal schedule preparing for a performance in 1 month. She is new to on-point toe dancing, beginning 8 months ago, and had some initial bilateral foot and knee pain but this has resolved in the past 6 months. She is anxious about missing dance rehearsals, which may jeopardize her role in the upcoming performance.

REVIEW OF SYSTEMS
The patient's ROS is positive for fatigue, generalized achiness, and recent history of fever (high of 102.5°F prior night) associated with sore throat presumptive for strep. Her sore throat is nearly resolved. The patient reports intermittent non-pruritic rash on her chest and bilateral arms and legs. She denies joint changes, except left knee pain, stiffness, swelling, and redness. She denies prior rashes, especially any bulls-eye lesion, and has had no known tick bites. The ROS is negative for weight loss, chills, eye pain, redness, discharge, ear pain, nasal congestion, cough, SOB, wheezing or sputum, chest pain, or palpitations. The patient denies nausea, vomiting, diarrhea, constipation, or changes in appetite or diet. She has not yet started her menses and denies urinary frequency, urgency, hematuria, dysuria, or vaginal discharge. No symptoms of joint pain or swelling beyond left knee noted. She appears mildly anxious and has had some difficulty sleeping due to knee discomfort and concern about return to dance activities; she denies depression. Her appetite is normal, and she maintains a good weight despite a heavy exercise schedule with dance. Confidentially, the patient denies sexual activity, risk to sexually transmitted infections, anorexia, or bulimia.

RELEVANT HISTORY
The patient's father states the child is generally healthy. She was full-term pregnancy with normal delivery at 39 weeks. She has had a history of typical childhood illnesses and achieved normal developmental milestones. No prior history of similar joint swelling or rashes. No serious or chronic illness. No surgeries, hospitalizations, accidents, or injuries. Immunizations are up to date. No prior reactions to medications or immunizations. The patient lives at home with her mother, father, sister, and brother in rural community. She attends public middle school and does well with grades. She attends dance rehearsal three times weekly. The family enjoys hiking and camping in a Lyme disease tick-endemic area. Her family history is negative for arthritis, systemic lupus, or IBD.

ALLERGIES

No known drug allergies; no known food allergies.

MEDICATIONS

- Amoxicillin 250 mg PO TID, for 6 days.
- Acetaminophen 500 mg PO last night and this morning, for fever, achiness, and knee pain.

PHYSICAL EXAMINATION

Vitals: T 38.3°C (101.0°F), P 88, R 16, BP 98/64, WT 39.25 kg (86.5 lbs), HT 147 cm (58 in.), BMI 18.1.

General: Alert, oriented, cooperative, mildly anxious voicing concerns about return to dance.

Psychiatric: Non-depressed appearing.

Skin, Hair, and Nails: Macular erythematous to salmon colored non-blanching rash scattered over upper torso and upper extremities, no sandpaper texture, no urticaria. Face, palms, and soles clear. No petechiae or ecchymosis noted. No abnormal findings with hair or nails.

Eyes: No redness, swelling, or discharge.

ENT/Mouth: No facial pain. TM clear. Positive light reflex, landmarks, mobility. No nasal drainage or oral lesions. Throat is mildly red; 2+ tonsils bilaterally, no exudate.

Neck: FROM, no rigidity.

Lymphatic: Lymph nodes 2+ non-tender anterior cervical chain bilaterally. Axillary and groin nodes non-enlarged.

Lungs: Clear without rales, rhonchi, or wheezes.

Heart: RRR without murmur, rubs, gallops, or bruits.

Abdomen: Non-tender, non-distended, without hepatosplenomegaly.

Peripheral vascular: Bilateral lower extremity distal pedal pulses normal (3+), capillary refill time <2 seconds (<3 seconds for normal pediatrics).

Musculoskeletal: Mild limp left knee with weight bearing. Left knee is warm, erythematous with generalized swelling and mild flexion reduction due to discomfort and edema. No evidence of trauma; skin is intact without lesions. No localized tenderness with palpation; no increased anterior/posterior, lateral, or patellar discomfort or joint line tenderness. Stress range of motion deferred due to discomfort. Palpations of distal femur, tibia, and fibula are non-tender without mass. Ballottement produces patellar bogginess suggestive of effusion. No additional joints involved. Hips with full range of motion without discomfort.

Neurologic: Cranial nerves II to XII grossly intact. Bilateral lower extremities without paresthesia.

CLINICAL DISCUSSION QUESTIONS

1. What is the differential diagnosis?

_____

_____

_____

2. What is the most likely diagnosis? Why?

_____

_____

_____

_____

3. Demonstrate your understanding about the pathophysiology in regard to the most likely diagnosis.

_____

_____

_____

_____

4. Should tests/imaging studies be ordered? Which ones? Why? Think about tests/imaging beyond the primary care setting as well.

_____

_____

_____

_____

5. What are the next appropriate steps in management?

_____

_____

_____

_____

6. Demonstrate your understanding of typical presentation, treatments, and complications of the diagnosis. Also investigate the adverse effects the diagnosis may cause on families. Include your references.

_____

_____

_____

_____

7. What are the pertinent ICD-10 and CPT (E/M) codes for this visit? Provide a short rationale.

_____

_____

_____

_____

8. What are the appropriate patient and parent education topics for this case?

_____

_____

_____

_____

9. If not managed appropriately, what is/are the medical/legal concern(s) that may arise?

_____

_____

_____

_____

10. Think about interprofessional collaboration for this case. Provide a list of specialties or other disciplines and indicate what contribution these professionals might make to managing the patient.

_____

_____

_____

_____

BEDSIDE MANNER QUESTION

11. What would your communication style/approach be with this patient and parent?

_____

_____

_____

_____

ANSWER KEY _available at_
https://connect.springerpub.com/content/book/978-0-8261-8273-9

WIDESPREAD PAINFUL RASH, PEDIATRIC FEMALE

CHIEF COMPLAINT

"Widespread painful rash."

HISTORY OF PRESENT ILLNESS

A mother and her 9-year-old daughter present to a pediatric clinic for a second opinion regarding the daughter's symptoms of fever, sore throat, and a painful rash. She had been seen 3 days earlier by her regular PCP, who diagnosed a viral infection. Her parents were concerned and sought a second opinion because she had a persistent high fever and her rash had worsened. The rash had extended to her extremities, had multiple areas of blistering, and continued to be painful. Within the past 24 hours, she developed sores on her lips and purulent discharge from both eyes. She is currently on day 9 of antibiotic treatment for uncomplicated cystitis.

Ten days prior to this visit, she had seen her regular PCP for evaluation of dysuria. She had no fever at that time. She was diagnosed with cystitis and prescribed a course of sulfamethoxazole-trimethoprim. The dysuria resolved within 24 hours and did not recur. Five days after starting the antibiotic, she developed a fever up to 40°C (104°F), generalized malaise, a mild sore throat, and skin pain. On day 6 of antibiotic treatment, she developed a rash on her face and trunk and was seen again by her PCP. Her parents stated that the rash was deep red and consisted of irregular blotchy areas with one or two small blisters. Her parents were told that her symptoms were most likely due to a viral infection because she was already taking an antibiotic.

They were advised to continue the antibiotic as prescribed and to give acetaminophen PRN for fever. No follow-up was scheduled.

REVIEW OF SYSTEMS

The patient's ROS is positive for generalized weakness, decreased appetite, eye pain, and photophobia. Her ROS is negative for headache, neck pain, vomiting, diarrhea, or abdominal pain.

RELEVANT HISTORY

The patient's history is significant for several episodes of otitis media, one previous episode of cystitis about 2 years earlier, and two episodes of streptococcal pharyngitis since starting kindergarten. There is no history of chronic illness. Her immunizations are up to date for age.

ALLERGIES

No known drug allergies; no known food allergies.

MEDICATIONS

- Sulfamethoxazole-trimethoprim 400 mg/80 mg PO BID.
- Acetaminophen 325 mg PO QID PRN for pain.

PHYSICAL EXAMINATION

Vitals: T 39.6°C (103.3°F), P 96, R 18, BP 92/56 mmHg, HT 127 cm (50 in.), WT 28.2 kg (62 lbs), BMI 17.4.

General: Ill appearing, in moderate discomfort.

Skin, Hair, and Nails: Face, trunk, and extremities with extensive erythematous and dark purple irregularly shaped macules with overlying vesicles of varying sizes (up to approximately 3 to 4 cm in diameter) and areas of deep skin erosion covering a small percentage of total skin surface; skin tender to light touch. No abnormal findings with hair or nails.

Head: No scalp lesions.

Eyes: Moderate conjunctival injection with small amount of purulent discharge bilaterally.

ENT/Mouth: Tympanic membranes translucent with normal mobility, oropharynx with mild erythema, lips erythematous with several areas of erosion and crusting.

Neck: FROM without discomfort; no resistance to flexion; no lymphadenopathy.

Lungs: Clear to auscultation bilaterally.

Heart: RRR, S1 and S2 normal intensity, no murmurs or extra heart sounds.

Abdomen: Soft, non-tender; no mass or hepatosplenomegaly.

Genital/Rectal: No lesions of external genitalia.

Musculoskeletal: No joint swelling, full range of motion.

Neurologic: Responds appropriately to questions; cranial nerves intact; strength and sensation not assessed due to skin lesions and tenderness; walks but appears to be in pain with movement.

CLINICAL DISCUSSION QUESTIONS

1. What is the differential diagnosis?

_____

_____

_____

_____

_____

2. What is the most likely diagnosis? Why?

_____

_____

_____

_____

_____

3. Demonstrate your understanding of the pathophysiology in regard to the most likely diagnosis.

_____

_____

_____

_____

_____

4. Should tests/imaging studies be ordered? Which ones? Why? Think about tests/imaging beyond the primary care setting as well.

_____

_____

_____

_____

_____

5. What are the next appropriate steps in management?

_____

_____

_____

_____

_____

6. What are the causes, risk factors, and treatment for this diagnosis? Provide references for your responses.

_____

_____

_____

_____

_____

7. What are the pertinent ICD-10 and CPT (E/M) codes for this visit? Provide a short rationale.

_____

_____

_____

_____

8. What are appropriate parent/patient education topics for this case?

_____

_____

_____

_____

_____

9. If not managed appropriately, what is/are the medical/legal concern(s) that may arise?

_____

_____

_____

_____

10. Think about interprofessional collaboration for this case. Provide a list of specialties or other disciplines and indicate what contribution these professionals might make to managing the patient.

_____

_____

_____

_____

_____

BEDSIDE MANNER QUESTIONS

11. What would your communication style/approach be with this mother and patient?

_____

_____

_____

_____

12. If a patient and her mother are distressed by the diagnosis, what might offer support?

_____

_____

_____

_____

ANSWER KEY *available at*
https://connect.springerpub.com/content/book/978-0-8261-8273-9

BLURRED VISION IN THE LEFT EYE, ADULT FEMALE

CHIEF COMPLAINT

"Blurred vision in the left eye."

HISTORY OF PRESENT ILLNESS

A 63-year-old Caucasian woman with a history of hypertension, diabetes, and myopia presents to her PCP with an acute onset of blurred vision in the left eye. She stated that it seemed like "a curtain came down over my eye" and was progressively getting worse by the time she arrived at the clinic. She was wearing dark glasses to relieve the discomfort from sunlight. Prior to her blurred vision, she experienced flashes of light and floaters in the eye. The patient was anxious and worried about permanent vision loss.

REVIEW OF SYSTEMS

A ROS is positive for blurred vision, flashes, floaters, and mild photophobia in the left eye. Her ROS is negative for pain, double vision, halos, or eye redness. She denies fever, chills, headaches, diarrhea, vomiting, or weight change. The patient denies other HEENT symptoms such as hearing defects and nostril or sinus problems. Her cardiopulmonary systems were unremarkable. She has no chest pain, SOB palpitations, or extremity edema. A neurologic ROS is negative for dizziness, confusion, gait imbalances, or extremity weakness.

RELEVANT HISTORY

The patient has a history of hypertension (diagnosed at age 50 and well controlled by lifestyle and antihypertensives). She has a history of poorly controlled type 2 diabetes (diagnosed at age 55) and was taking oral antidiabetic drugs, (last A1C was 7.8). Other medical conditions included myopia diagnosed during her childhood. She denies any history of recent trauma, illness, or hospitalization except for cataract surgery 2 years ago. The patient is a retired postal worker, married, and living with her husband in a senior housing condominium. She quit smoking cigarettes at age 40 and reports occasional use of alcohol (about one glass of wine weekly). She is on a DASH diet with regular exercises through a support group from her church.

ALLERGIES

Penicillin (skin rash); no known food allergies.

MEDICATIONS

- Metformin 850 mg BID.
- Hydrochlorothiazide/lisinopril 12.5 mg/20 mg QD.
- Atorvastatin 10 mg QHS.
- Over-the-counter multivitamin.

PHYSICAL EXAMINATION

Vitals: T 37°C (98.6°F), P 90, R 16, BP 135/80, WT 90 kg (198.4 lbs), HT 170 cm (66.9 in.), BMI 32.9.

General: Well-developed and nourished Caucasian woman in no acute distress. She appears mildly anxious but alert and oriented to person, place, time, and situation.

Skin, Hair, and Nails: Skin was fair, warm, and moist with good skin turgor. No jaundice, erythema, rashes, or scales noted. There are no signs of nodularity, thickening, or pain on skin palpation. Hair and nails showed no abnormal findings.

Head: She has no lesions, scaling, or scalp tenderness.

Eyes: Vision is reduced bilaterally (20/30 in the right eye; blurred in left eye but able to count fingers at 3 feet); pupils were reactive to light. Extraocular movements are full, but patient has both temporal and nasal visual field deficits in the left eye. Tonometry measuring of intraocular pressure (IOP): 17 mmHg in the right eye and 12 mmHg in the left eye.

ENT/Mouth: Ears, nares, mouth, and throat have no abnormal findings.

Neck: Supple with no cervical adenopathy or thyroid enlargement.

Lungs: Respiratory rate is 16 and un-labored. Trachea is midline. She has normal A-P diameter. No tenderness on palpation. Tactile fremitus and respiratory expansion are normal. The lungs are clear to auscultation. No wheezes, crackles, or rhonchi bilaterally.

Heart: RRR, without murmur, gallop, or rub.

Peripheral Vascular: Dorsalis pedis and posterior tibial pulses are faint (1/4).

Neurologic: Alert and oriented. Most cranial nerves are intact. Sensation and reflexes are present in all extremities.

CLINICAL DISCUSSION QUESTIONS

1. What is the differential diagnosis?

_____

_____

_____

_____

2. What is the most likely diagnosis? Why?

_____

_____

_____

_____

3. Demonstrate your understanding about the pathophysiology in regard to the most likely diagnosis.

_____

_____

_____

_____

4. Should tests/imaging studies be ordered? Which ones? Why? Think about tests/imaging beyond the primary care setting as well.

_____

_____

_____

_____

5. What are the next appropriate steps in management?

_____

_____

_____

_____

6. Review recent and credible research articles on about this diagnosis. Demonstrate your understanding of the diagnostic criteria, supplemental testing, and treatment approach. Provide references with your response.

_____

_____

_____

_____

7. What are the pertinent ICD-10 and CPT (E/M) codes for this visit? Provide a short rationale.

_____

_____

_____

_____

8. What is the appropriate patient education topics for this case?

_____

_____

_____

_____

9. If not managed appropriately, what is/are the medical/legal concern(s) that may arise?

_____

_____

_____

_____

10. Think about interprofessional collaboration for this case. Provide a list of specialties or other disciplines and indicate what contribution these professionals might make to managing the patient.

_____

_____

_____

_____

BEDSIDE MANNER QUESTION

11. What would your communication style/approach be with this patient?

_____

_____

_____

_____

ANSWER KEY _available at_
https://connect.springerpub.com/content/book/978-0-8261-8273-9

FEVER AND BACK PAIN, GERIATRIC FEMALE

CHIEF COMPLAINT
"Fever and back pain."

HISTORY OF PRESENT ILLNESS
A 78-year-old woman presents to her regular PCP with a 2-day history of fatigue, malaise, and fever. She awoke this morning with a dull ache in her right mid-back and some nausea. She came to the office because she is concerned about the pain and her worsening symptoms. She has been resting and taking acetaminophen (650 mg every 4 to 6 hours), which has helped with the fever and aches, but her symptoms return as the drug wears off. She is unsure of how high her fever has gotten. She states the pain is a 3 or 4 out of 10, but the fatigue, malaise, and nausea have kept her from her daily activities and caused her to stay in bed most of yesterday and today. She believes she might have "the flu" though she received the vaccine 3 weeks ago. She is most concerned because she lives alone and is afraid of becoming seriously ill and having no way to call for help. She denies ever smoking and drinks a glass of wine only once or twice a month. Her husband of many years died 8 years ago of prostate cancer, and she lives independently in an apartment. One of her three children lives a few miles away and visits frequently. She is not currently sexually active.

She denies chills, night sweats, rhinorrhea, cough, SOB, dyspnea, chest pains, palpitations, vomiting, diarrhea, or constipation. She admits to increased urinary frequency and urgency but denies pain with urination. She denies sick contacts or changes to her dietary routine.

REVIEW OF SYSTEMS
The patient's ROS is positive for occasional knee pain. Her ROS is negative for weakness, weight loss, focal pain except in the right flank, difficulty with memory or concentration, recent illness, or injury.

RELEVANT HISTORY
The patient's history is significant for hypertension and osteoporosis. She has a family history of CAD. Her daughter lives nearby and is available to stay with her if needed.

ALLERGIES
No medication, environmental, or food allergies.

MEDICATIONS
- Lisinopril/hydrochlorothiazide 10/12.5 mg daily.
- Alendronate 70 mg weekly.
- OTC 1,000 mg calcium citrate with 600 IU vitamin D3 daily.

PHYSICAL EXAMINATION

Vitals: T 38.8°C (101.8°F), P 96, R 14, BP 106/68, WT 56.7 kg (125 lbs), HT 172.72 cm (68 in.), BMI 20.2.

General: Ill and uncomfortable appearing, but non-toxic and without acute distress.

Psychiatric: Alert and oriented to person, place, and time; coherent conversation.

Skin, Hair, and Nails: Skin pale and slightly flushed, no rash or lesion. Nails are smooth without hemorrhage.

Eye: Eyes without retinal lesions.

ENT/Mouth: Oral mucosa moist without lesions.

Chest: Symmetric excursion with no accessory muscle use.

Breasts: No mass or lesion bilaterally.

Lungs: Resonant with vesicular breath sounds all fields; no wheezes, rales, or rhonchi.

Heart: Quiet precordium; RSR; no murmur, rub, or gallop.

Abdomen: Flat, normoactive bowel sounds all quadrants, no mass. There is mild right costovertebral angle tenderness and mild suprapubic discomfort but no tenderness.

Genital/Rectal: Vaginal and introital mucosa show atrophy. The uterus is small and smooth. No mass or lesion detected in the adnexa or cul-de-sac.

Musculoskeletal: No point tenderness detected on the vertebral processes.

CLINICAL DISCUSSION QUESTIONS

1. What is the differential diagnosis?

_____

_____

_____

_____

2. What is the most likely diagnosis? Why?

_____

_____

_____

_____

3. Demonstrate your understanding about the pathophysiology in regard to the most likely diagnosis.

_____

_____

_____

_____

4. Should tests/imaging studies be ordered? Which ones? Why? Think about tests/imaging beyond the primary care setting as well.

_____

_____

_____

_____

5. What are the next appropriate steps in management?

_____

_____

_____

_____

6. Review a recent and credible research article about the key factors (causes, risks, diagnostic testing, and treatment selection) of this diagnosis. Provide references for your response.

_____

_____

_____

_____

7. What are the pertinent ICD-10 and CPT (E/M) codes for this visit? Provide a short rationale.

_____

_____

_____

_____

8. What is the appropriate patient education for this case?

_____

_____

_____

_____

9. If not managed appropriately, what is/are the medical/legal concern(s) that may arise?

_____

_____

_____

10. Think about interprofessional collaboration for this case. Provide a list of specialties or other disciplines and indicate what contribution these professionals might make to managing the patient.

_____

_____

_____

_____

BEDSIDE MANNER QUESTION

11. What would your communication style/approach be with this patient?

_____

_____

_____

_____

ANSWER KEY _available at_
https://connect.springerpub.com/content/book/978-0-8261-8273-9

SORE THROAT, FEVER, AND CHILLS, ADULT MALE

CHIEF COMPLAINT

"Sore throat, fever, and chills."

HISTORY OF PRESENT ILLNESS

A 25-year-old man with a history of asthma and diabetes presents as a new patient with a 4-day history of a sore throat that had worsened overnight. His throat initially started hurting 4 to 5 days ago; however, he now has associated subjective fever, chills, and pain upon swallowing. The pain is burning, constant, rated 8/10, and it radiates to his left ear. He has been taking ibuprofen the last 4 days without significant relief. The patient has had sore throats prior to this episode, but he has "never had pain like this before." Previous episodes typically occurred with symptoms of a "cold" and lasted 1 to 2 days. He is able to tolerate soft foods and liquids. He is accompanied today by his father.

REVIEW OF SYSTEMS

The patient's ROS is positive for fever, chills, odynophagia, trismus, and otalgia. His ROS is negative for malaise, fatigue, nausea, vomiting, cough, SOB, hemoptysis, abdominal pain, neck pain, and rash.

RELEVANT HISTORY

The patient's relevant history is positive for type 2 diabetes and asthma, both well controlled. He is married and has one daughter. He denies tobacco use, drinks "a few" beers on the weekend, smokes marijuana on occasion, and denies other recreational drugs. His father is well, with chronic, uncomplicated diabetes and hypertension. His mother is alive and well with chronic hypertension complicated by chronic kidney disease.

ALLERGIES

No known drug allergies; no known food allergies.

MEDICATIONS

- Albuterol inhaler two puffs inhaled, q4h to q6h PRN.
- Metformin 500 mg PO BID.

PHYSICAL EXAMINATION

Vitals: T 38.1°C (100.5°F), P 103, R 18, BP 132/78, SpO$_2$ 99%, 90.72 kg (200 lbs), 182.88 cm (72 in.), BMI 27.12.

General: Ill-appearing male sitting on the bed, in mild distress related to pain. Patient is speaking in short sentences, and his voice is muffled and low pitch in quality.

Psychiatric: Cooperative, mildly anxious secondary to pain.

Skin, Hair, and Nails: No rashes or abnormal pigmentation noted. No abnormal findings with hair or nails.

Head: Atraumatic, normocephalic.

Eyes: Conjunctiva pink and moist, PEERLA, EOMI.

ENT/Mouth: Bilateral TM intact, pearly gray in color, cone of light noted, serous fluid appreciated on the left; no erythema or exudates noted. Mucosa pink and moist; no lesions, swelling, or drainage noted in nose. Difficulty opening his mouth. Buccal mucosa slightly dry; posterior pharynx is erythematous; mild white tonsillar exudate bilateral, (2+) tonsillar enlargement on the right, (3+) tonsillar enlargement on the left, and deviation of the uvula toward the right noted.

Neck: Supple, no bruits appreciated, trachea midline, no thyromegaly appreciated, lymphadenopathy noted with tender to palpation at site of the left submandibular region and along the left superficial cervical chain.

Lungs: Normal A/P diameter; non-labored breathing; symmetric chest wall expansion; no chest wall tenderness to palpation; breath sounds clear to auscultation bilaterally, without wheezing, rales, or rhonchi.

Heart: RRR, S1 and S2 present (normal); no murmurs, rubs, or gallops.

Abdomen: Non-distended, positive BS, soft, non-tender; no masses or splenomegaly appreciated.

Neurologic: Alert and oriented to person, time, and place. Cranial nerves II to XII grossly intact.

CLINICAL DISCUSSION QUESTIONS

1. What is the differential diagnosis?

_____

_____

_____

_____

2. What is the most likely diagnosis? Why?

_____

_____

_____

_____

3. Demonstrate your understanding about the pathophysiology in regard to the most likely diagnosis.

_____

_____

_____

_____

4. Should tests/imaging studies be ordered? Which ones? Why? Think about tests/imaging beyond the primary care setting as well.

_____

_____

_____

_____

5. What are the next appropriate steps in management?

_____

_____

_____

6. What are the risk factors and predictors for hospitalization for the diagnosis? Provide references for your response.

_____

_____

_____

_____

7. What are the pertinent ICD-10 and CPT (E/M) codes for this visit? Provide a short rationale.

_____

_____

_____

_____

8. What is the appropriate patient education for this case?

_____

_____

_____

_____

9. If not managed appropriately, what is/are the medical/legal concern(s) that may arise?

_____

_____

_____

_____

10. Think about interprofessional collaboration for this case. Provide a list of specialties or other disciplines and indicate what contribution these professionals might make to managing the patient.

_____

_____

_____

_____

BEDSIDE MANNER QUESTIONS

11. What would your communication style/approach be with this patient and his father?

_____

_____

_____

_____

12. If a patient and his father are distressed by the diagnosis, what might offer support?

_____

_____

_____

_____

ANSWER KEY _available at_
https://connect.springerpub.com/content/book/978-0-8261-8273-9

BAD COUGH AND FEVER, ADOLESCENT FEMALE

CHIEF COMPLAINT

"Bad cough and fever."

HISTORY OF PRESENT ILLNESS

A 14-year-old girl is brought to her PCP's office by her mother in December for evaluation of a cough for 5 days and fever for 2 days with a maximum temperature at home of 103.1°F (39.5°C), tympanic, last night. Her symptoms began with nasal congestion and sore throat 5 days ago along with a mild cough that has progressed over the last 48 hours to become productive and more severe and with two episodes of post-tussive emesis. The patient occasionally is short of breath and complains of chills.

REVIEW OF SYSTEMS

The patient's ROS is positive for malaise, intermittent headache, nasal congestion, rhinorrhea, sore throat, cough, and occasional dyspnea, post-tussive emesis, fever, chills, and chest pain with cough. The ROS is negative for vision or hearing disturbances, otalgia, neck pain or stiffness, wheezing, nausea, diarrhea, constipation, abdominal pain, rash, urinary symptoms, or arthralgia.

RELEVANT HISTORY

The patient's medical history is unremarkable and negative for any known medical conditions. She has never been hospitalized and has no known drug allergies. Her immunizations are up to date for her age, including an influenza vaccine 3 months ago. She began her menses about a year ago She is in the 9th grade at a public school and an average student. She states, "Everybody at school is sick."

ALLERGIES

No known drug allergies; no known food allergies.

MEDICATIONS

- Acetaminophen 325 mg tablets—two every 4 to 6 hours PRN. Last dose was 4 hours ago.
- An OTC cough medicine she does not recall the name of. The mother thinks it is a generic Robitussin DM. It is not helping.

PHYSICAL EXAMINATION

Vitals: T 39.0°C (102.2°F), P 102, R 24, BP 120/76, SpO$_2$ 95% on room air, WT 58 kg (129 lbs), HT 165 cm (65 in.), BMI 21.5 (about 75th percentile).

General: Ill appearing with frequent coughing but no acute distress.

Psychiatric: Normal mood and affect.

Eyes: Sclerae clear.

ENT/Mouth: Nasal mucosa shows boggy edema with scant mucopurulent drainage bilaterally. Mouth mucosa pink and moist with mild posterior pharyngeal erythema. There is no sinus tenderness to facial percussion.

Neck: Supple with firm, mobile, and fingertip-sized bilateral non-tender lymphadenopathy.

Lungs: No accessory muscle use with good air movement. There are diffuse moist rhonchi and end-expiratory wheezes at the bases. There is dullness to percussion in the lower lung fields.

Heart: RRR, with normal S1 and S2. No murmurs, rubs, or gallops.
Abdomen: Normal bowel sounds, soft and nontender; no organomegaly.
Neurologic: A&O×3.

CLINICAL DISCUSSION QUESTIONS

1. What is the differential diagnosis?

_____

_____

_____

_____

2. What is the most likely diagnosis? Why?

_____

_____

_____

_____

3. Demonstrate your understanding about the pathophysiology in regard to the most likely diagnosis.

_____

_____

_____

_____

4. Should tests/imaging studies be ordered? Which ones? Why? Think about tests/imaging beyond the primary care setting as well.

_____

_____

_____

_____

5. What are the next appropriate steps in management?

_____

_____

_____

_____

6. What is the prevalence in this patient population? What are the diagnostic challenges and treatment options for this diagnosis? Provide references for your responses.

_____

_____

_____

7. What are the pertinent ICD-10 and CPT (E/M) codes for this visit? Provide a short rationale.

_____

_____

_____

_____

8. What is the appropriate patient education for this case?

_____

_____

_____

_____

9. If not managed appropriately, what is/are the medical/legal concern(s) that may arise?

_____

_____

_____

_____

10. Think about interprofessional collaboration for this case. Provide a list of specialties or other disciplines and indicate what contribution these professionals might make to managing the patient.

_____

_____

_____

_____

BEDSIDE MANNER QUESTIONS

11. What would your communication style/approach be with this patient and her mother?

_____

_____

_____

_____

12. If a patient and her mother are distressed by the diagnosis, what might offer support?

_____

_____

_____

_____

ANSWER KEY *available at*
https://connect.springerpub.com/content/book/978-0-8261-8273-9

HEADACHE AND FEVER, PEDIATRIC MALE

CHIEF COMPLAINT

"Headache and fever."

HISTORY OF PRESENT ILLNESS

An 8-year-old boy is brought to his pediatric office for a rapidly worsening headache and fever. Parents report he had been in a good state of health and returned about 5 days ago from a week at a scout camp. They deny any recent head injury. There have been no known tick bites. On the last day, he began to feel tired and developed a headache and fever. The maximum fever they obtained at home was 103.2°F. His appetite has been steadily declining over the past 10 hours or so. They tried ibuprofen, and it helped the headache initially but no longer seems to give relief. He denies cough, congestion, sore throat, diarrhea, or rash. He has vomited once in the past 30 minutes. Over the past 2 hours, he has not been himself. He doesn't want to move, wants the lights out, and is less interactive. He moans and complains of head and neck pain. The nurse informs the PCP that the boy is not speaking clearly when she asks him questions and is confused. She has tried to find out where the headache localizes to but he cannot offer that information at this time. He cannot explain severity either. The nurse feels this patient requires immediate attention.

REVIEW OF SYSTEMS

His ROS was positive for headache, fever, confusion, neck pain, vomiting, anorexia, and nausea. His ROS is negative for cough, congestion, sore throat, rash, or diarrhea. He denies dysuria, hematuria, and abdominal pain. No wheezing or SOB is noted.

RELEVANT HISTORY

Patient has a history of exercise-induced asthma that is well controlled with the use of his albuterol inhaler prior to activities. He takes no other medication or supplements. He has no prior surgery history. He has no allergies to medication, and his vaccinations are up to date. He lives with his mother and father in an apartment that was built in the last 5 years. His only recent travel was the scout camp. The paternal history is positive for IBS. The maternal history is positive for hypothyroidism diagnosed at the age of 21.

ALLERGIES

No known drug or food allergies.

MEDICATIONS

Albuterol inhaler 1–2 puffs inhaled x1: start 5–30 minutes before exercise.

PHYSICAL EXAMINATION

Vitals: T 40°C (104°F), P 115, R 22, BP 102/68, WT 30.2 kg (66.5 lbs), HT 137.2 cm (54 in.), BMI 16.

General: Ill appearing. Moans and cries at times. Answers some questions but seems confused about where he is currently.

Skin, Hair, and Nails: Warm and dry. Few scattered petechiae are noted on the lower extremities that were not noted in nurse documentation. These lesions are not blanchable. No peripheral edema. No jaundice. No abnormal findings with hair and nail exam.

Head: Normocephalic. Atraumatic with no bruising noted.

Eyes: Refuses eye exam and cries, "The light is too bright." Pupils appear equal and reactive. Cannot assess extraocular muscles at this time.

ENT/Mouth: TMs are pearly bilaterally with no erythema or effusion. Nares are patent with no congestion. Oropharynx is somewhat dry but without erythema or exudate.

Neck: Very tender to palpation. Patient refuses to bend neck forward and cries in pain if attempted. Flexion at the hips occurs when forcibly attempted. This is noted as a positive Brudzinski sign. Mild scattered anterior cervical adenopathy. Nodes mobile and not firm. No thyromegaly.

Lungs: Clear to auscultation bilaterally. No wheezes or crackles. Good aeration noted throughout. No stridor.

Heart: RRR with no murmur noted.

Abdomen: Soft. Cries with palpation but doesn't localize to a single area. No rebound. No guarding. Bowel sounds normal throughout all fields. Non-distended.

Genital/Rectal: Normal Tanner 1 on exam. Rectal exam deferred.

Musculoskeletal: Patient is non-cooperative for thorough exam. Will not stand up from bed for exam secondary to neck pain and headache. Muscle strength appears equal in the upper and lower extremities bilaterally at likely 4/5. Attempts to move hips in to a flexed position and then extend the lower legs while laying flat are met with intense resistance and moans of pain. This is a positive Kernig sign.

Neurologic: Patient is non-cooperative for thorough exam. Will not stand up from bed for exam secondary to neck pain and headache. Will not cooperate to check cranial nerves secondary to pain in neck and head; appear intact. Attempts to check deep tendon reflexes are met with cries when he has to move. Incomplete exam but appears to have reflexes of +3/5 in the upper and lower extremities that are symmetric.

CLINICAL DISCUSSION QUESTIONS

1. What is the differential diagnosis?

_____

_____

_____

_____

2. What is the most likely diagnosis? Why?

_____

_____

_____

_____

3. Demonstrate your understanding about the pathophysiology in regard to the most likely diagnosis.

_____

_____

_____

_____

4. Should tests/imaging studies be ordered? Which ones? Why? Think about tests/imaging beyond the primary care setting as well.

_____

_____

_____

_____

5. What are the next appropriate steps in management?

_____

_____

_____

_____

6. What are physical exam findings, treatment approach, causes, and prevention of the diagnosis? Provide references for your response.

_____

_____

_____

_____

7. What are the pertinent ICD-10 and CPT (E/M) codes for this visit? Provide a short rationale.

_____

_____

_____

_____

8. What is the appropriate patient education for this case?

_____

_____

_____

_____

9. If not managed appropriately, what is/are the medical/legal concern(s) that may arise?

_____

_____

_____

_____

10. Think about possible interprofessional collaboration in this case. Provide a list of names and indicate their contribution to managing the patient.

_____

_____

_____

_____

BEDSIDE MANNER QUESTIONS

11. What would your communication style/approach be with this patient and his parents?

_____

_____

_____

_____

12. If a patient and his parents are distressed by the diagnosis, what might offer support?

_____

_____

_____

_____

ANSWER KEY *available at*
https://connect.springerpub.com/content/book/978-0-8261-8273-9

HEART PALPITATIONS, ADULT FEMALE

CHIEF COMPLAINT

"Heart palpitations."

HISTORY OF PRESENT ILLNESS

A 64-year-old woman presents to her regular PCP complaining of chest palpitations. She was watching TV and suddenly her heart started racing and pounding. She became light-headed and felt a bit better after a while. She reports she hears her heart beating when lying down. She is concerned and now presents for evaluation. She reports having mild palpitations in the past but nothing like this. She has a history of atrial fibrillation and was taken off her blood thinners by her urologist and oncologist. She was diagnosed with kidney cancer 5 months ago and is now 4 months post right nephrectomy. She denies any chest pain or syncope. She reports she never refilled her previous medication and she did not follow up with her PCP post-surgery.

REVIEW OF SYSTEMS

The patient's ROS is positive for chest palpitations, generalized weakness, and SOB. Her ROS is negative for weight loss or gain, fever, chills, vomiting, diarrhea, constipation, and chest pain.

RELEVANT HISTORY

This patient has a history of hypertension, renal cancer, coronary artery disease, GERD, and a systolic murmur. She also has a new lung lesion. Her surgical history is positive for a nephrectomy 4 months ago. The patient is a widow and lives with her only child, an unmarried son. She denies tobacco use, alcohol use, or any illicit drug use. She has a family history of CAD, hypertension, and type 2 diabetes, but no family history of cancer.

ALLERGIES

No known drug allergies; no known food allergies.

MEDICATION

- Diltiazem 180 mg PO QD (empty pill bottle).
- Lisinopril 20 mg PO QD.
- Metoprolol succinate 50 mg QD (empty pill bottle).
- Low-dose aspirin, 81 mg PO QD.

PHYSICAL EXAMINATION

Vitals: T 36.8°C (98.3°F), P 130, R 18, BP 110/74, WT 80.7 kg (178 lbs), HT 160 cm (63 in.), BMI 31.5.

General: Lethargic but not in acute distress.

Psychiatric: Smiles; is cooperative and answers all questions appropriately though slightly slow to respond but states this is her baseline after the nephrectomy and her surgeon said it is to be expected.

Lungs: Nonlabored, chest rise symmetrical, lungs clear upon auscultation bilaterally.

Heart: Irregular rhythm and rapid heart rate, systolic murmur right sternal border grade 3/6.

Neurologic: Alert and awake (GCS = 15), but delayed verbal response; motor and sensory is intact; deep tendon reflex 2+ bilaterally; Romberg is negative.

CLINICAL DISCUSSION QUESTIONS

1. What is the differential diagnosis?

_____

_____

_____

_____

2. What is the most likely diagnosis? Why?

_____

_____

_____

3. Demonstrate your understanding about the pathophysiology in regard to the most likely diagnosis.

_____

_____

_____

_____

4. Should tests/imaging studies be ordered? Which ones? Why? Think about tests/imaging beyond the primary care setting as well.

_____

_____

_____

_____

5. What are the next appropriate steps in management?

_____

_____

_____

_____

6. What are the prevalence, incidence, and complications of the diagnosis? Provide references for your responses.

_____

_____

_____

_____

7. What are the pertinent ICD-10 and CPT (E/M) codes for this visit? Provide a short rationale.

_____

_____

_____

_____

8. What is the appropriate patient education for this case?

_____

_____

_____

_____

9. If not managed appropriately, what is/are the medical/legal concern(s) that may arise?

_____

_____

_____

_____

10. Think about interprofessional collaboration for this case. Provide a list of specialties or other disciplines and indicate what contribution these professionals might make to managing the patient.

_____

_____

_____

_____

BEDSIDE MANNER QUESTION

11. What would your communication style/approach be with this patient?

_____

_____

_____

_____

ANSWER KEY *available at*
https://connect.springerpub.com/content/book/978-0-8261-8273-9

DOUBLE AND BLURRED VISION, ADOLESCENT MALE

CHIEF COMPLAINT

"Double and blurred vision."

HISTORY OF PRESENT ILLNESS

A 15-year-old boy, accompanied by his mother, presents to a new PCP with a 2-week history of double and blurred vision. He has not had any prior episodes. He reports he noticed it first while during physical education class. The episodes last about 5 to 10 minutes each time. Over the past 2 weeks, he recalls having about 10 episodes. He reports that resting relieves his symptoms. They tend to be worse the longer he is physically active or if he is having a particularly stressful day. He reports having occasional headaches; however, he denies headache currently. When the headaches occur, he describes them as throbbing with pain behind both eyes. He denies SOB and chest pain.

REVIEW OF SYSTEMS

The patient's ROS is positive for fatigue, double and blurred vision, and occasional headaches. He denies current headache or vision changes. The patient reported past dizziness and light-headedness; he has not had any syncope. He denies being dizzy at the time of exam. His ROS is negative for fever, chills, palpitations, heat or cold intolerance, SOB, edema, or chest pain. His weight has been stable, and he denies any heat or cold intolerance.

RELEVANT HISTORY

The patient's history is positive for obesity. His mother reports that previous health providers had expressed concern about his elevated blood pressure. She does not recall the blood pressure readings, but was told on more than one occasion that they were elevated. According to previous health care providers, he attempted lifestyle changes but failed. The patient has no other medical history. His immunizations are up to date. He lives with his parents and 7-year-old sister. He reports enjoying school; he is a sophomore and enjoys reading and hanging out with his friends. He has a relatively sedentary lifestyle; he exercises only when required in his gym class. His family history is positive for his mother with hypertension and type 2 diabetes; his father has hyperlipidemia and reports having "borderline" high blood pressure. His sister is healthy. Maternal grandparents are unknown; his mother was adopted. Paternal grandfather is deceased, but had a history of stroke, MI, and hypertension; he passed away from a second stroke at age 60. Paternal grandmother, age 73, is alive and obese with hypertension, type 2 diabetes, and hyperlipidemia.

ALLERGIES

No known drug allergies; no known food allergies.

MEDICATIONS

None.

PHYSICAL EXAMINATION

Vitals: T 36.7°C (98.2°F); P 90; R 16; BP 138/86; HT 175.26 cm (69 in.), ~75th percentile for age; WT 80.164 kg (180 lbs); BMI 26.6, 95th percentile for his age.

General: Appears calm in no acute distress. Obese, appears to be stated age.

Psychiatric: Calm and cooperative.

Skin, Hair, and Nails: Skin intact, no tenting or rashes noted. No abnormal findings with hair or nails.

Head: Normocephalic, no deformities noted.

Eyes: PERRLA. Vision 20/20 with both eyes.

Neck: Supple, FROM, no thyromegaly noted.

Lungs: Clear to auscultation in all lung fields.

Heart: RRR. No murmurs, rubs, or gallops noted.

Musculoskeletal: FROM in all extremities, no edema or deformities noted.

Neurologic: The patient is alert, attentive, and oriented. Speech is clear and fluent.

Cranial nerves: II—Visual fields are full to confrontation; funduscopic exam is normal with sharp discs and no vascular changes; pupils are 4 mm and briskly reactive to light; visual acuity is 20/20 bilaterally. III, IV, VI—There is no eye deviation; convergence is impaired; PERRLA. V—Facial sensation is intact; corneal reflexes are intact. VII—Face is symmetric. VIII—Hearing is normal to rubbing fingers and whisper test. IX, X—Palate elevates symmetrically; phonation is normal. XI—Head turning and shoulder shrug are intact. XII—Tongue is midline with normal movements and no atrophy. Motor: There is no pronator drift of out-stretched arms; no atrophy noted; strength 5/5 bilaterally. Reflexes: 2+ and symmetric in the bilateral upper and lower extremities; sensory is intact bilaterally. Coordination: There are no abnormal or extraneous movements; Romberg is negative. Gait/stance: Posture is normal; gait is steady.

CLINICAL DISCUSSION QUESTIONS

1. What is the differential diagnosis?

_____

_____

_____

_____

2. What is the most likely diagnosis? Why?

_____

_____

_____

_____

3. Demonstrate your understanding about the pathophysiology in regard to the most likely diagnosis.

_____

_____

_____

_____

4. Should tests/imaging studies be ordered? Which ones? Why? Think about tests/imaging beyond the primary care setting as well.

_____

_____

_____

_____

5. What are the next appropriate steps in management?

_____

_____

_____

_____

6. What are the risk factors, diagnostic criteria, and treatment options of the diagnosis? Provide references for your response.

_____

_____

_____

_____

7. What are the pertinent ICD-10 and CPT (E/M) codes for this visit? Provide a short rationale.

_____

_____

_____

_____

8. What are the appropriate patient and parent education topics for this case?

_____

_____

_____

_____

9. If not managed appropriately, what is/are the medical/legal concern(s) that may arise?

_____

_____

_____

_____

10. Think about interprofessional collaboration for this case. Provide a list of specialties or other disciplines and indicate what contribution these professionals might make to managing the patient.

_____

_____

_____

_____

BEDSIDE MANNER QUESTION

11. What would be your communication style/approach with this patient and parent?

_____

_____

_____

_____

ANSWER KEY _available at_
https://connect.springerpub.com/content/book/978-0-8261-8273-9

NIPPLE PAIN, ADULT FEMALE

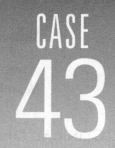

CHIEF COMPLAINT
"Nipple pain."

HISTORY OF PRESENT ILLNESS
A 34-year-old Caucasian woman presents to her PCP with a 3-day history of pain in her right nipple. She presents to the appointment alone and is a good historian. She is married, the mother of two children ages 3 years and 9 months, and is a part-time loan officer at a local bank. She is currently breastfeeding and began to wean the infant about 1 week ago. She generally breastfeeds at night and pumps for daytime feedings. Three days ago, she experienced sharp shooting pains in the right nipple with some radiation to the right axilla. She described the pain as 6/10 on 0–10 pain scale. She has tried white willow bark, cool compresses, and breast massage for letdown of milk without any success. Today, she presents with continued complaints of right nipple pain, some malaise, headache, and "not feeling well."

REVIEW OF SYSTEMS
The patient's ROS is positive for breast pain with radiation, low-grade fever, and malaise. Her ROS is negative for breast lump, erythema, or nipple discharge, sleep disturbance, irritability or sadness, numbness, or tingling.

RELEVANT HISTORY
The patient is generally healthy with no major health problems. Her obstetric history is G2 P2 normal spontaneous vaginal delivery, with both deliveries born at home at term with midwife assistance. No postpartum difficulties. Both children were breastfed.

ALLERGIES
No known drug allergies; no known food allergies.

MEDICATIONS
None.

PHYSICAL EXAMINATION
Vitals: T 37.9°C (100.2°F), P 76, R 20, BP 118/64, WT 55.3 kg (122 lbs), HT 165.1 cm (65 in.), BMI 20.5.

General: In mild discomfort. Appears fatigued.

Psychiatric: Affect is normal and appropriate.

Lungs: Respirations even and un-labored, clear bilaterally.

Heart: Normal S1, S2 without rubs, murmurs, or gallops.

Right Breast: Full without engorgement. Mild pain to palpation of nipple radiating to 3 o'clock location and right axilla. Mild breast erythema noted. No nipple discharge without stimulation; upon stimulation able to obtain specimen.

Musculoskeletal: Motor 5/5 proximal and distal upper extremities, including shoulders. DTRs 2+ and symmetrical of knees, brachioradialis, and biceps tendons. Bilateral upper grips equal and strong. No pain with ROM.

Neurologic: A&O×3, cranial nerves II to XII grossly intact.

CLINICAL DISCUSSION QUESTIONS

1. What is the differential diagnosis?

_____

_____

_____

_____

2. What is the most likely diagnosis? Why?

_____

_____

_____

_____

3. Demonstrate your understanding about the pathophysiology in regard to the most likely diagnosis.

_____

_____

_____

_____

4. Should tests/imaging studies be ordered? Which ones? Why? Think about tests/imaging beyond the primary care setting as well.

_____

_____

_____

_____

5. What are the next appropriate steps in management?

_____

_____

_____

_____

6. What are the causing pathogens and treatment options for this diagnosis? Provide references for your response.

_____

_____

_____

_____

7. What are the pertinent ICD-10 and CPT (E/M) codes for this visit? Provide a short rationale.

_____

_____

_____

_____

8. What is the appropriate patient education for this case?

_____

_____

_____

_____

9. If not managed appropriately, what is/are the medical/legal concern(s) that may arise?

_____

_____

_____

_____

10. Think about interprofessional collaboration for this case. Provide a list of specialties or other disciplines and indicate what contribution these professionals might make to managing the patient.

_____

_____

_____

_____

BEDSIDE MANNER QUESTION

11. What would your communication style/approach be with this patient?

_____

_____

_____

_____

ANSWER KEY *available at*
https://connect.springerpub.com/content/book/978-0-8261-8273-9

IRREGULAR MENSTRUAL CYCLE, ADOLESCENT FEMALE

CHIEF COMPLAINT

"Irregular menstrual cycle."

HISTORY OF PRESENT ILLNESS

A 17-year-old young woman presents to her PCP with a 1-year history of irregular menses, including skipped menses, menorrhagia, and dysmenorrhea. She presents to the appointment with her mother, who assists as historian. She started menarche at age 14 and states she has never really had regular menses. Over the past year, menses have increased in irregularity and flow with clots, with menstrual cramping. Menses are 7 days in length with mild to moderate clots. Patient uses tampons and changes them during menses, hourly for the first 3 to 4 days and then every 3 hours for the last 2 to 3 days of her menses. The patient states that about twice a year she does not have a menses and related that this is usually during a time of excess physical activity and stress.

REVIEW OF SYSTEMS

The patient's ROS is positive for nausea, abdominal pain (menstrual cramping), heavy menstrual flow, and intermittent dizziness. Her ROS is negative for decrease in appetite, weight change, hair loss, vaginal discharge, depression, or fatigue.

RELEVANT HISTORY

The patient has no history of depression or eating disorders and no history of chronic medical problems or surgery. She lives with parents and siblings in a single-family home. She takes advanced placement classes in school in the 12th grade at the local high school. The patient is active in school and community sports, including dance, volleyball, and soccer. She has been very involved with sports in middle and high school. Her family history is positive for thyroid disorders and hypertension but negative for bleeding disorders. She denies being sexually active. She denies any eating disorder tendencies. She denies any usage of tobacco, alcohol, and drugs.

ALLERGIES

No known drug allergies; no known food allergies.

MEDICATIONS

None.

PHYSICAL EXAMINATION

Vitals: T 37°C (98.7°F); P 98; R 22; BP 108/62; WT 55.34 kg (122 lbs), 50th percentile; HT 165 cm (65 in.), 60th percentile; BMI 20.

General: Appears mildly fatigued.

Psychiatric: Affect is normal and appropriate.

Head: Head is normocephalic. Hair distribution is normal without hair loss.

Eyes: PERRL, red reflex present bilaterally. EOM full, positive nystagmus.

ENT/Mouth: Tympanic membranes pearly gray with visible cone of light and landmarks. Mucosa is pink and moist. Normal speech and tone. Uvula midline.

Neck: Neck supple, no thyromegaly, or adenopathy.

Lungs: Respirations even and un-labored, clear bilaterally.

Heart: Normal S1 S2 without rubs, murmurs, or gallops.

Abdomen: Soft, non-tender, BS ×4, no organomegaly or splenomegaly. No costovertebral angle tenderness.

Musculoskeletal: Moves all extremities well, equal strength, gait normal, DTRs 2+ bilaterally.

Neurological: A&O×3, cranial nerves II to XII grossly intact. Sensory grossly intact to light touch symmetrically.

CLINICAL DISCUSSION QUESTIONS

1. What is the differential diagnosis?

_____

_____

_____

_____

2. What is the most likely diagnosis? Why?

_____

_____

_____

_____

3. Demonstrate your understanding about the pathophysiology in regard to the most likely diagnosis.

_____

_____

_____

_____

4. Should tests/imaging studies be ordered? Which ones? Why? Think about tests/imaging beyond the primary care setting as well.

_____

_____

_____

_____

5. What are the next appropriate steps in management?

_____

_____

_____

_____

6. Review a credible article(s) about environmental factors and characteristics of menarche associated with the diagnosis. Provide your references.

_____

_____

_____

_____

7. What are the pertinent ICD-10 and CPT (E/M) codes for this visit? Provide a short rationale.

_____

_____

_____

_____

8. What is the appropriate patient education for this case?

_____

_____

_____

_____

9. If not managed appropriately, what is/are the medical/legal concern(s) that may arise?

_____

_____

_____

_____

10. Think about interprofessional collaboration for this case. Provide a list of specialties or other disciplines and indicate what contribution these professionals might make to managing the patient and parent.

_____

_____

_____

_____

BEDSIDE MANNER QUESTIONS

11. What would your communication style/approach be with this patient and mother?

_____

_____

_____

_____

12. If the patient and her mother are distressed by the diagnosis, what might offer support?

_____

_____

_____

_____

ANSWER KEY _available at_
https://connect.springerpub.com/content/book/978-0-8261-8273-9

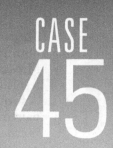

RIGHT KNEE PAIN, PEDIATRIC FEMALE

CHIEF COMPLAINT
"Right knee pain."

HISTORY OF PRESENT ILLNESS
A 10-year-old girl accompanied by her mother presents to her pediatric office with right knee pain. Her pain started approximately 4 weeks ago and is getting progressively worse. She denies any initial injury. Generally, it is always bothering her but gets worse with activities. She is unable to run as fast as she wants due to the pain, which interferes with her sports. She has pain after practices. She reports the knee is better with ibuprofen, when resting and when icing. The pain is sharp with activities but dull otherwise. The pain does not radiate. The pain is limiting her activities. She plays soccer and volleyball. She has had practice most days of the week for the last 6 weeks. The patient rates her pain as 7/10.

REVIEW OF SYSTEMS
The ROS is positive for joint pain, gait problem with exercise, and swelling of the lower leg. The ROS is negative for weight loss, fever, dyspnea on exertion, orthopnea, chest pain, rash, warmth to touch, numbness, or decreased ROM of any joints.

RELEVANT HISTORY
The patient denies any history of surgeries or hospitalizations. Her immunizations are up to date. She demonstrates normal growth and development. The patient takes no daily medications but uses loratadine PRN for seasonal allergies. She has no exposure to tobacco use.

ALLERGIES
No known drug allergies; allergic to shrimp.

MEDICATIONS
Ibuprofen 200 mg, every 6 hours as needed for pain.

PHYSICAL EXAMINATION
Vitals: T 37.2°C (99°F), P 90, R 16, BP 100/80, WT 46.50 kg (102.5 lbs), HT 152.4 cm (60 in.), BMI 20.

General: Well-developed and nourished female appearing age appropriate.

Psychological: Normal mood and affect.

Skin, Hair, and Nails: Warm and dry, no rashes noted. No abnormal findings with hair or nails.

Lungs: Clear to auscultation bilaterally.

Heart: RRR with no murmurs or extra heart sounds.

Musculoskeletal: Inspection of knee revealed no ecchymosis, rash, or laceration. Left knee FROM both actively and passively. Palpation revealed Lachman, anterior and posterior drawer tests, and McMurray test are negative. Right knee has FROM both actively and passively. Apprehension test is negative bilateral. There are no joint effusions on bilateral knees. The right tibial tuberosity is swollen compared to the left. The right tibial tuberosity is exquisitely tender to the touch; no pain on the left. There is no warmth or erythema to the swelling. Bilateral hip and ankle joints are normal.

Neurologic: A&O×3. DTRs are 2+ bilaterally patellar. Strength is 5/5 for the lower extremities.

CLINICAL DISCUSSION QUESTIONS

1. What is the differential diagnosis?

_____

_____

_____

_____

2. What is the most likely diagnosis? Why?

_____

_____

_____

3. Demonstrate your understanding about the pathophysiology in regard to the most likely diagnosis.

_____

_____

_____

_____

4. Should tests/imaging studies be ordered? Which ones? Why? Think about tests/imaging beyond the primary care setting as well.

_____

_____

_____

_____

5. What are the next appropriate steps in management?

_____

_____

_____

6. What are the risk factors, treatment options, and prognosis of the diagnosis? Provide references for your response.

_____

_____

_____

_____

7. What are the pertinent ICD-10 and CPT (E/M) codes for this visit? Provide a short rationale.

_____

_____

_____

_____

8. What is the appropriate patient education for this case?

_____

_____

_____

_____

9. If not managed appropriately, what is/are the medical/legal concern(s) that may arise?

_____

_____

_____

_____

10. Think about interprofessional collaboration for this case. Provide a list of specialties or other disciplines and indicate what contribution these professionals might make to managing the patient.

_____

_____

_____

_____

BEDSIDE MANNER QUESTIONS

11. What would your communication style/approach be with this patient and her mother?

_____

_____

_____

_____

12. If a patient and her mother are distressed by the diagnosis, what might offer support?

_____

_____

_____

_____

Answer Key _available at_
https://connect.springerpub.com/content/book/978-0-8261-8273-9

CHEST PAIN, ADOLESCENT MALE

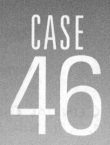

CHIEF COMPLAINT
"Chest pain."

HISTORY OF PRESENT ILLNESS
A 14-year-old otherwise healthy boy presents with his mother to his PCP complaining of right-sided chest pain, which began 1 day ago after he sustained an injury playing football. The patient states he was playing tackle football with friends when he received an injury to the right side of his chest from a player's elbow. He immediately fell to the ground in pain. He lay still for 1 to 2 minutes, expecting the pain to subside, but it did not. He attempted to continue playing but experienced difficulty taking a deep breath and the pain was more noticeable when running and twisting. The patient took 600 mg of ibuprofen the night before, but the medication did not relieve his pain. After a restless night, his mother has brought him for evaluation.

REVIEW OF SYSTEMS
The patient's ROS is positive for SOB, chest pain, decreased range of motion of torso due to pain, and bruising after an injury. The patient is negative for fever, vision changes, loss of consciousness, cough, palpitations, edema, nausea, vomiting, diarrhea, numbness, and tingling.

RELEVANT HISTORY
The boy's medical history is unremarkable. His immunizations are up to date, he has no surgical history, and he takes no medications. He lives with his mother, father, and 10-year-old sister. He denies alcohol, tobacco, or illicit drug use. The family history is non-contributory.

ALLERGIES
No known drug allergies; no known food allergies.

MEDICATIONS
Ibuprofen 600 mg PRN for pain.

PHYSICAL EXAMINATION
Vitals: T 37.7°C (99.8°F), P 102, R 24, BP 124/76, SpO$_2$ 98%, WT 61.90 kg (136.5 lbs), HT 162.5 cm (64 in.), BMI 23.6.

General: Appears in acute distress.

Psychiatric: Mildly anxious.

Skin, Hair, and Nails: No rash; skin warm and dry. No abnormal findings with hair or nails.

Chest: Bruising and tenderness to palpation of right lateral chest wall located in mid-axillary line at approximately the 4th and 5th intercostal spaces. No pain with lateral rotation of torso. Pain elicited with forward flexion and extension of the torso. Symmetrical movement of chest wall with inspiration and expiration.

Lungs: Clear to auscultation bilaterally with diminished breath sounds in right lower lobe. Percussion to posterior chest wall on right demonstrates hyperresonance.

Heart: RRR; no murmurs, rubs, or gallops.

Abdomen: Soft, non-tender, non-distended. No hepatosplenomegaly. Positive bowel sounds in all four quadrants.

Neurologic: A&O×3, with no focal motor or sensory deficits noted.

CLINICAL DISCUSSION QUESTIONS

1. What is the differential diagnosis?

_____

_____

_____

_____

2. What is the most likely diagnosis? Why?

_____

_____

_____

_____

3. Demonstrate your understanding about the pathophysiology in regard to the most likely diagnosis.

_____

_____

_____

_____

4. Should tests/imaging studies be ordered? Which ones? Why? Think about tests/imaging beyond the primary care setting as well.

_____

_____

_____

_____

5. What are the next appropriate steps in management?

_____

_____

_____

_____

6. Review a reliable and recent article and discuss the treatment approach for this diagnosis. Include the reference.

_____

_____

_____

_____

7. What are the pertinent ICD-10 and CPT (E/M) codes for this visit? Provide a short rationale.

_____

_____

_____

_____

8. What are appropriate patient education topics for this case?

_____

_____

_____

_____

9. If not managed appropriately, what is/are the medical/legal concern(s) that may arise?

_____

_____

_____

_____

10. Think about interprofessional collaboration for this case. Provide a list of specialties or other disciplines and indicate what contribution these professionals might make to managing the patient.

_____

_____

_____

_____

Bedside Manner Questions

11. What would your communication style/approach be with this patient and his mother?

_____

_____

_____

12. If a patient and his mother are distressed by the diagnosis, what might offer support?

_____

_____

_____

_____

ANSWER KEY available at
https://connect.springerpub.com/content/book/978-0-8261-8273-9

RECURRENT PAIN AND REDNESS IN LEFT FOOT, ADULT FEMALE

CHIEF COMPLAINT

"Recurrent pain and redness in left foot."

HISTORY OF PRESENT ILLNESS

A 36-year-old woman presents to her PCP with increased pain in her left foot. The pain has been present for the past 3 months but has gotten worse the past week. She also complains of an intermittent low-grade fever and chills. Her fever comes and goes but is present mainly at night. She states that 6 months ago she had a similar episode and was seen at an urgent care, where antibiotics were prescribed, and her pain subsided. Today, she complains the pain has been gradually increasing and her lower left leg is warm to touch and red. The pain and swelling increase with activity. Elevating and resting the foot decrease the pain and swelling but they return as soon as she resumes activity. She denies any injury or trauma to her left leg or foot.

REVIEW OF SYSTEMS

The patient's ROS is positive for a low-grade fever, chills, left foot swelling, redness, and pain to left foot. The patient reported malaise and fatigue and pain and redness to left foot. Her ROS is negative for nausea, vomiting, decreased appetite, chest pain, or SOB. She denies hip or knee pain. She denies any recent injury or trauma.

RELEVANT HISTORY

The patient has type 2 diabetes and hypertension (age 28). Six months ago, she developed a wound over the left ankle and foot that is now closed. The patient is a smoker of 1 pack of cigarettes/day. She is single and lives alone with her two dogs and three cats. Her family history includes diabetes and hypertension.

ALLERGIES

No known drug allergies; no known food allergies.

MEDICATIONS

- Metformin 1,000 mg BID.
- Enalapril 10 mg QD.

PHYSICAL EXAMINATION

Vitals: T 38.1°C (100.6°F), P 82, R 20, BP 128/82, WT 68 kg (150 lbs), HT 165 cm (65 in), BMI 24.2.

General: Alert and cooperative. Sitting comfortably on the exam table. Does not have a toxic or distressed appearance. Well hydrated, well nourished.

Skin, Hair, and Nails: Skin warm and dry. Rest of the exam within normal findings.

Neck: Supple with FROM and no lymphadenopathy present.

Lungs: Clear to auscultation bilaterally. No rales or rhonchi present.

Heart: RRR. Normal S2.

Musculoskeletal: At the left ankle and foot, diffuse blanching erythema and trace nonpitting edema noted. At the dorsum of the left foot and anterolateral aspect of the talofibular joint, there is a 3×3 cm^2 area of erythema and warmth, tender to palpation. ROM full to ankle.

Neurologic: Left foot with normal sensation and 2+ pedal pulse to posterior tibia and dorsalis pedis. No drop foot present.

CLINICAL DISCUSSION QUESTIONS

1. What is the differential diagnosis?

_____

_____

_____

_____

2. What is the most likely diagnosis? Why?

_____

_____

_____

_____

3. Demonstrate your understanding about the pathophysiology in regard to the most likely diagnosis.

_____

_____

_____

_____

4. Should tests/imaging studies be ordered? Which ones? Why? Think about tests/imaging beyond the primary care setting as well.

_____

_____

_____

_____

5. What are the next appropriate steps in management?

_____

_____

_____

_____

6. What is the treatment approach for this diagnosis? Provide references for your response.

_____

_____

_____

_____

7. What are the pertinent ICD-10 and CPT (E/M) codes for this visit? Provide a short rationale.

_____

_____

_____

_____

8. What is the appropriate patient education for this case?

_____

_____

_____

_____

9. If not managed appropriately, what is/are the medical/legal concern(s) that may arise?

_____

_____

_____

_____

10. Think about interprofessional collaboration for this case. Provide a list of specialties or other disciplines and indicate what contribution these professionals might make to managing the patient.

_____

_____

_____

_____

BEDSIDE MANNER QUESTION
11. What would your communication style/approach be with this patient?

_____

_____

_____

_____

ANSWER KEY *available at*
https://connect.springerpub.com/content/book/978-0-8261-8273-9

MUSCLE AND JOINT PAIN, ADULT FEMALE

CHIEF COMPLAINT
"Muscle and joint pain."

HISTORY OF PRESENT ILLNESS
A 45-year-old woman presents to her PCP with muscle and joint pain. She complains of fatigue, headache, neck stiffness, and poor appetite. She returned to California last night from Rhode Island, where she had been on a summer camping trip with several close friends. She camped 2 days at the beginning of her 10-day trip in Rhode Island. She denies fever, chills, nausea, vomiting, constipation, abdominal pain, cough, runny nose, sore throat, ear pain, nasal congestion, rash, dysuria, urinary urgency, SOB or chest pain. She is married and her husband went camping with her. She does not recall seeing any ticks while camping. She denies having a tick bite. However, she recalls one of her friends screamed that she saw a tick on her lower leg. When asked for more information about her husband, she states he is doing well but just tired from the long trip. When asked if he had seen any ticks during the camping, she states, "He didn't mention anything like that." When asked if her husband has any rash, she states, "Yes. He noticed ringworm this morning and applied some topical cream." She states her husband gets ringworm occasionally from their dog.

REVIEW OF SYSTEMS
The patient's ROS is positive for muscle pain, joint pain, neck stiffness, and anorexia. She reports fatigue and headache. Her ROS is negative for fever, chills, nausea, vomiting, constipation, abdominal pain, cough, runny nose, sore throat, ear pain, nasal congestion, rash, dysuria, urinary urgency, SOB and chest pain.

RELEVANT HISTORY
The patient's history is significant for hypothyroidism (onset age 30), benign hypertension (onset age 35), hypercholesteremia (onset age 30), and obesity. She had two Cesarean sections. She has had no other surgery. Her social history includes traveling with her husband. She has been working as a referral clerk for a healthcare clinic. She has one sister and one brother. She has been sexually active (no protection) since age 20 with her husband and they are in a monogamous relationship. Her family history includes diabetes, MI and CAD (father) and breast cancer, hypothyroidism, and diabetes (mother). Her family history is negative for autoimmune disease.

ALLERGIES
No known drug allergies; no known food allergies.

MEDICATIONS
- Levothyroxine 50 mcg daily.
- Hydrochlorothiazide/lisinopril 12.5 mg/10 mg daily.
- Atorvastatin 20 mg daily.

PHYSICAL EXAMINATION

Vitals: T 37.2°C (99.0°F), P 78, R 18, BP 130/86, HT 162.6 cm (64 in.), WT 73.9 kg (163 lbs), BMI 28.

General: No acute distress, communicates well, afebrile.

Psychiatric: Appropriate mood and affect.

Skin, Hair, and Nails: No skin rash or lesion appreciated. No abnormal findings with hair or nails.

Eyes: Conjunctiva and sclera clear, no injection or exudate.

ENT/Mouth: Ear canals clear, TMs pearly gray, intact with normal light reflex. No nasal deformity, pharynx without erythema or exudate.

Lungs: Clear to auscultation, good air movements throughout.

Heart: RRR, no murmurs, radial and femoral pulses strong and equal.

Abdomen: Soft, non-tender, not distended.

Lymphatic: Palpable lymph nodes on cervical, axillary (bilateral), and inguinal (bilateral).

Musculoskeletal: Muscle strength appropriate and equal bilaterally, full range of active and passive motion; muscle tenderness noted; generalized.

Neurologic: A&O×3, cranial nerves II to XII intact.

CLINICAL DISCUSSION QUESTIONS

1. What is the differential diagnosis?

_____

_____

_____

_____

2. What is the most likely diagnosis? Why?

_____

_____

_____

_____

3. Demonstrate your understanding about the pathophysiology in regard to the most likely diagnosis.

_____

_____

_____

_____

4. Should tests/imaging studies be ordered? Which ones? Why? Think about tests/imaging beyond the primary care setting as well.

_____

_____

_____

_____

5. What are the next appropriate steps in management?

_____

_____

_____

_____

6. Review a reliable, recent source and discuss screening labs, diagnosis criteria, and treatment plans for the diagnosis. Provide references for your responses.

_____

_____

_____

_____

_____

7. What are the pertinent ICD-10 and CPT (E/M) codes for this visit? Provide a short rationale.

_____

_____

_____

_____

8. What is the appropriate patient education for this case?

_____

_____

_____

_____

9. If not managed appropriately, what is/are the medical/legal concern(s) that may arise?

_____

_____

_____

_____

10. Think about interprofessional collaboration for this case. Provide a list of specialties or other disciplines and indicate what contribution these professionals might make to managing the patient.

_____

_____

_____

_____

BEDSIDE MANNER QUESTION

11. What would your communication style/approach be with this patient?

_____

_____

_____

_____

ANSWER KEY *available at*
https://connect.springerpub.com/content/book/978-0-8261-8273-9

CONSTIPATION, ADOLESCENT FEMALE

CHIEF COMPLAINT

"Constipation."

HISTORY OF PRESENT ILLNESS

A 17-year-old young woman presents to her PCP with complaints of persistent constipation for about 6 months. Her mother is present and confirms her daughter often complains of feeling full after just a few bites of food, abdominal discomfort and bloating, and difficulty passing bowel movements. The patient admits she does not always drink enough water through her day but eats a balanced diet and tries to stay active. Her mother reports having tried polyethylene glycol for her daughter "a few times" with some benefit but no other interventions. On further discussion, the patient does admit that it has been harder for her to be active lately as she always feels tired. She is a runner and a swimmer but notes her performance in both sports has declined and she feels "slow" and "blah" most days. Her mother reports she sleeps about 7 to 8 hours per night, does not recall her snoring or gasping for breath, and denies hearing her wake often at night. The patient denies being overly anxious or depressed and reports good social activity. She is doing well in school, behaves appropriately at home, and works part-time at a pizzeria with good work behaviors. Her only other concern is a 7-lb weight gain over the past few months despite having decreased appetite but states, "I just thought it was because I wasn't going to the bathroom enough."

REVIEW OF SYSTEMS

The patient's ROS is positive for constipation, abdominal discomfort and bloating, weight gain, and fatigue. Her ROS is negative for vomiting or diarrhea, blood in stools, fever, and chills. She denies changes in her menstrual cycle. Her ROS is negative for chest pain or palpitations, SOB, dizziness or headache, and anxiety or depression. No hair or skin changes are noted, as well as no joint pain or swelling.

RELEVANT HISTORY

The patient had a fracture of 5th metatarsal of right foot at age 12; her last menstrual period was 2 weeks ago. She attends 11th grade in a public school with As and Bs in all classes. She denies smoking (including vaping), drinking, or alcohol use. She lives at home with her mother and a younger brother. Parents are divorced but her father is very active in her life and supportive. She denies sexual activity and has no history of STIs. Her vaccinations and preventive screening are up to date and unremarkable. Her family history is significant for mother with hypothyroidism and paternal grandfather with type 2 diabetes.

ALLERGIES

No known drug allergies; no known food allergies.

MEDICATIONS

Polyethylene glycol 3350 PRN.

PHYSICAL EXAMINATION

Vitals: T 36°C (96.8°F); P 68; R 14; BP 108/64; WT 68 kg (150 lbs), increased from 65 kg (143 lbs) last visit 3 months ago; HT 157.5 cm (62 in.); BMI 24.2.

General: A&O×3, well groomed.

Psychiatric: Normal affect, pleasant, and cooperative.

Skin, Hair, and Nails: Skin dry but without rash or lesions. No abnormal findings with hair or nails.

Neck: Supple with some mild thyromegaly, no nodules. No cervical lymph nodes.

Lungs: Clear to auscultation with normal respiratory effort.

Heart: S1 S2 RRR; no murmur noted.

Abdomen: Mild distention with firmness and mild tenderness on palpation. Stool detected in descending colon.

Rectal: Hard stool in rectal vault noted but no blood. No internal or external hemorrhoids; negative for occult blood.

Musculoskeletal: No redness or swelling of joints, with FROM.

Neurologic: Patellar DTRs 1+ bilaterally (mildly diminished), normal gait and station. Cranial nerves grossly intact.

CLINICAL DISCUSSION QUESTIONS

1. What is the differential diagnosis?

_____

_____

_____

_____

2. What is the most likely diagnosis? Why?

_____

_____

_____

_____

3. Demonstrate your understanding about the pathophysiology in regard to the most likely diagnosis.

_____

_____

_____

_____

4. Should tests/imaging studies be ordered? Which ones? Why? Think about tests/imaging beyond the primary care setting as well.

_____

_____

_____

_____

5. What are the next appropriate steps in management?

_____

_____

_____

_____

6. What are the different types of organ dysfunction (primary organ associated with the case) and what is the role of autoimmune diseases of this diagnosis? Provide references for your responses.

_____

_____

_____

_____

7. What are the pertinent ICD-10 and CPT (E/M) codes for this visit? Provide a short rationale.

_____

_____

_____

_____

8. What is the appropriate patient education for this case?

_____

_____

_____

_____

9. If not managed appropriately, what is/are the medical/legal concern(s) that may arise?

_____

_____

_____

_____

10. Think about interprofessional collaboration for this case. Provide a list of specialties or other disciplines and indicate what contribution these professionals might make to managing the patient.

_____

_____

_____

_____

BEDSIDE MANNER QUESTIONS

11. What would be your communication style/approach with this patient and her mother?

_____

_____

_____

_____

12. If a patient and her mother are distressed by a diagnosis, what might offer support?

_____

_____

_____

_____

ANSWER KEY _available at_
https://connect.springerpub.com/content/book/978-0-8261-8273-9

COUGHING AND WHEEZING, PEDIATRIC MALE

CHIEF COMPLAINT

"Coughing and wheezing."

HISTORY OF PRESENT ILLNESS

A 6-year-old boy presents with his mother to a new PCP with a 6-week history of coughing and wheezing. He has not had routine well-child checks due to several relocations, but he is up to date on vaccines and his mother would like to establish care. His mother says the coughing and wheezing have been steadily worsening over the past several weeks during winter season but are significantly worse in the past 2 weeks. He coughs throughout the daytime and wakes up several times at night during the week. In the past week, he has used his albuterol inhaler daily for cough/wheeze, and sometimes it is so bad that he "can't breathe." He has gone to the ED twice in the past year for coughing and wheezing, was given nebulized breathing treatments with significant improvement of symptoms, and was subsequently discharged home with an albuterol inhaler, 5 days of oral steroids, and instructions to follow up with the PCP. He has never required hospitalization. His mother says he is a very active child and loves to play soccer, but in the past 2 weeks, he has not been able to keep up with his teammates due to difficulty breathing while playing.

REVIEW OF SYSTEMS

ROS is positive for dry chronic cough, SOB and wheezing. The ROS is negative for fever, eye redness or discharge, nasal congestion/discharge, sneezing, earache, sore throat, decreased intake, decreased energy, decreased voids, change in stools, bulky/greasy stools, weight loss, night sweats, or rash.

RELEVANT HISTORY

The patient's past medical history is unremarkable except for the coughing and wheezing. There is no history of pneumonia, recurrent infections, seasonal allergies, or food allergies. TB skin test prior to starting kindergarten was negative last year. His mother smoked cigarettes during her pregnancy with this child and throughout his childhood until the present. He is in the 1st grade and has average performance, but he seems more distracted and impulsive in the past 2 months at school. He lives at home in an apartment with his mother and two older siblings (no pets). Parents had an amicable divorce 3 months ago and the patient sees his father every other weekend. Mother continues to smoke cigarettes but "only outside." Family history is significant for biologic father with asthma as a child.

ALLERGIES

No known drug allergies; no known food allergies.

MEDICATIONS

Albuterol inhaler 2 puffs every 4–6 hours PRN.

PHYSICAL EXAMINATION

Vitals: T 37.1°C (98.8°F); P 100; RR 24; BP 110/70; SpO$_2$ 97%; WT 22.7 kg (50 lbs), 75th percentile; HT 120 cm (47 in.), 75th percentile; BMI 15.8, 63rd percentile.

General: Well appearing, no acute distress, answering questions in complete sentences, talkative.

Skin, Hair, and Nails: Normal skin turgor, no rashes or dry patches. No abnormal findings with hair or nails.

Head: Normocephalic/atraumatic.

Eyes: EOM intact bilaterally, PERRLA bilaterally, no scleral injection, no eye discharge.

ENT: TMs normal bilaterally. Normal nasal turbinates bilaterally with pink mucosa, no discharge, normal pharynx. 2+ tonsils bilaterally without erythema, edema, or exudate.

Chest: Mild barrel chest, no retractions.

Lungs: End-expiratory wheeze diffusely in all anterior and posterior lung fields bilaterally, decreased air movement throughout.

Heart: RRR without murmur.

CLINICAL DISCUSSION QUESTIONS

1. What is the differential diagnosis?

_____

_____

_____

_____

2. What is the most likely diagnosis? Why?

_____

_____

_____

_____

3. Demonstrate an understanding of the pathophysiology of the most likely diagnosis.

_____

_____

_____

_____

4. Should tests/imaging studies be ordered? Which ones? Why? Think about tests/imaging beyond the primary care setting as well.

_____

_____

_____

_____

5. What are the next appropriate steps in management?

_____

_____

_____

_____

6. What are the risk factors, diagnostic studies, efficacy of medications, and medical costs associated with the diagnosis? Provide references for your responses.

_____

_____

_____

_____

7. What are the pertinent ICD-10 and CPT (E/M) codes for this visit? Provide a short rationale.

_____

_____

_____

_____

8. What are the appropriate patient education topics for this case?

_____

_____

_____

_____

9. If not managed appropriately, what is/are the medical/legal concern(s) that may arise?

_____

_____

_____

_____

10. Think about interprofessional collaboration for this case. Provide a list of specialties or other disciplines and indicate what contribution these professionals might make to managing the patient.

_____

_____

_____

_____

BEDSIDE MANNER QUESTIONS

11. What would your communication style/approach be with this patient?

_____

_____

_____

_____

ANSWER KEY *available at*
https://connect.springerpub.com/content/book/978-0-8261-8273-9

SHOULDER PAIN, ADULT MALE

CHIEF COMPLAINT
"Shoulder pain."

HISTORY OF PRESENT ILLNESS
A 48-year-old previously healthy, right-hand-dominant man presents with acute onset 8/10, deep, throbbing, non-radiating, right anterior shoulder pain for days. He denies trauma, history of same, lancinating pain, swelling, extremity weakness, and numbness/tingling. He reports he works as a firefighter and he recently participated in training exercises where he repeatedly "threw Molotov cocktails." He states he has been using ice and OTC ibuprofen every 8 hours without relief.

REVIEW OF SYSTEMS
The patient's ROS is positive for right shoulder pain. The ROS is negative for fever, skin changes/redness/bruising, joint pain, numbness, tingling, weakness, swelling, and trauma.

RELEVANT HISTORY
The patient's medical history is significant for hypertension (diagnosed age 43), currently controlled on HCTZ as well as chronic low back pain s/p L4/5 fusion (age 47). His social history includes occasional alcohol and marijuana use. He eats a balanced vegetarian diet and exercises for an hour daily. He is married with one son. His family history is positive for hypertension and hyperlipidemia in his father. His mother is well and healthy.

ALLERGIES
Penicillin (reaction: hives); no known food allergies.

MEDICATIONS
- 25 mg HCTZ daily
- OTC ibuprofen 200 mg 2 tablets q8h PRN

PHYSICAL EXAMINATION
Vitals: T 37.0°C (98.6°F), P 88, R 18, BP 138/92, HT 173 cm (68 in), WT 76.2 kg (168 lbs), BMI 25.7

General: Alert, no acute distress, non-toxic appearing.

Skin, Hair, and Nails: Right upper extremity: intact, no erythema, no ecchymosis, no abrasions/skin breakdown.

Head: Normocephalic, atraumatic.

Neck: FROM, no midline tenderness.

Lungs: Clear to auscultation bilaterally.

Heart: RRR, no murmurs, rubs, or gallops, radial pulse intact bilaterally, capillary refill <2 seconds.

Musculoskeletal: Right upper extremity: LROM to flexion, extension, internal and external rotation at shoulder due to pain, tender to palpation to anterior shoulder over insertion of long head of biceps, positive empty can test, negative cross-over test, no deformity, negative Hawkins, negative Neer, negative Apprehension test, 5/5 grip strength, no arm drop.

Neurologic: Sensation grossly intact to upper extremities.

CLINICAL DISCUSSION QUESTIONS

1. What is the differential diagnosis?

_____

_____

_____

_____

2. What is the most likely diagnosis? Why?

_____

_____

_____

3. Demonstrate your understanding about the pathophysiology in regard to the most likely diagnosis.

_____

_____

_____

_____

4. Should tests/imaging studies be ordered? Which ones? Why? Think about tests/imaging beyond the primary care setting as well.

_____

_____

_____

_____

5. What are the next appropriate steps in management?

_____

_____

_____

_____

6. What are the causes, physical exam techniques, and treatment options associated with this diagnosis? Provide references for your response.

_____

_____

_____

_____

7. What are the pertinent ICD-10 and CPT (E/M) codes for this visit? Provide a short rationale.

_____

_____

_____

_____

8. What is the appropriate patient education for this case?

_____

_____

_____

_____

9. If not managed appropriately, what is/are the medical/legal concern(s) that may arise?

_____

_____

_____

_____

10. Think about interprofessional collaboration for this case. Provide a list of specialties or other disciplines and indicate what contribution these professionals might make to managing the patient.

_____

_____

_____

_____

BEDSIDE MANNER QUESTION

11. What would your communication style/approach be with this patient?

_____

_____

_____

_____

PAINLESS ANAL BUMPS, ADULT TRANSGENDER MALE

CHIEF COMPLAINT

"Painless anal bumps."

HISTORY OF PRESENT ILLNESS

A 23-year-old transgender man presents to a new PCP with a several-month history of painless lesions around his anal area. He first noticed them while showering; they felt like little skin tags and were painless. Early on, he could only feel two or three. He states those are larger now, and more have emerged around the anus. He states they sometimes bleed after a bowel movement. He is sexually active with a self-identified gender non-conforming partner with male genitalia, and they engage in both vaginal and anal sex where the patient is the receptive partner. He denies any other history of STIs and gets regular HIV testing, and the last routine screens for HIV and STI testing at the local health department were negative.

The patient did see a local urgent care provider last week about his complaints. The clinician told him that they looked like skin tags, but might be warts, and if he waited, they should go away on their own. They have not, and this is why he has come to today's appointment.

REVIEW OF SYSTEMS

The patient's ROS is negative for any similar skin rashes on other areas of the body. He denies any vaginal or anal discharge or bleeding. He also denies any symptoms of fever, chills, changes in bowel habits, chest pain, abdominal pain, SOB, or any constitutional symptoms.

RELEVANT HISTORY

The patient's medical history is significant for elevated BP as told to him by a previous PCP, but he has never been diagnosed with hypertension and he takes no medications for this. His surgical history is significant for a tonsillectomy at age 18. He lives with his partner; they have been together for 2 years, and he denies other sexual partners. He states he has all his required vaccinations but does not remember if he had the HPV vaccine. He was asked to leave his parents' house at 19 when he embraced his gender identity and has not spoken with them since; they have all his childhood medical and vaccination records. His mental health is good, he sees a therapist regularly and has never been diagnosed with any formal psychological diagnoses.

We discussed his gender confirmation, a process he has embraced since he was a young teenager, but only began taking hormones 3 years ago when he became comfortable mentioning it to his medical provider. He reports no interest in a mastectomy as part of his confirmation at this point. He prefers to "go with the hormones" first before pursuing surgical interventions as well. In spite of the regular follow up, he states he has not had a full pelvic exam in years since his gender confirmation. Because none of his previous providers suggested he have one, he thought it was fine to just skip it.

He only takes injectable testosterone at this time, which he administers himself or sometimes his partner administers for him. His testosterone levels have ranged in the mid-400s, which he is happy with, and he has been pleased with facial hair growth, a deeper voice, and a notable increase in muscle mass. He has stopped having periods 2 years ago.

MEDICAL ALLERGIES

No known drug allergies; no known food allergies.

MEDICATIONS

Testosterone 200 mg IM every 2 weeks (he administers himself).

PHYSICAL EXAMINATION

Vitals: T 37.1°C (98.8°F), P 77, R 16, BP 128/84, WT 85.3 kg (188 lbs), HT 177.8 cm (70 in.), BMI 27.

General: Thin male in no apparent distress.

Genital/Rectal: Pelvic exam reveals unremarkable vaginal anatomy, no lesions or rashes noted, no cervical lesions or discharge noted. Rectal exam reveals multiple (>5) verruca-appearing lesions varying from 1 to 3 cm. No tenderness to palpation noted; no evidence of external bleeding. All lesions are immediately at the anal verge or immediately surrounding it, without evidence of outlet obstruction.

CLINICAL DISCUSSION QUESTIONS

1. What is the differential diagnosis?

_____

_____

_____

_____

2. What is the most likely diagnosis? Why?

_____

_____

_____

_____

3. Demonstrate your understanding about the pathophysiology in regard to the most likely diagnosis.

_____

_____

_____

_____

4. Should tests/imaging studies be ordered? Which ones? Why? Think about tests/imaging beyond the primary care setting as well.

_____

_____

_____

_____

5. What are the next appropriate steps in management?

_____

_____

_____

_____

6. Review a reliable, recent source and demonstrate an understanding of the prevalence, prevention, and treatments. Provide references for your responses.

_____

_____

_____

_____

7. What are the pertinent ICD-10 and CPT (E/M) codes for this visit? Provide a short rationale.

_____

_____

_____

_____

8. What is the appropriate patient education for this case?

_____

_____

_____

_____

9. If not managed appropriately, what is/are the medical/legal concern(s) that may arise?

_____

_____

_____

_____

10. Think about interprofessional collaboration for this case. Provide a list of specialties or other disciplines and indicate what contribution these professionals might make to managing the patient.

_____

_____

_____

_____

BEDSIDE MANNER QUESTIONS

11. What would your communication style/approach be with this patient?

_____

_____

_____

_____

12. If a patient is distressed by the diagnosis, what might offer support?

_____

_____

_____

_____

ANSWER KEY _available at_
https://connect.springerpub.com/content/book/978-0-8261-8273-9

FATIGUE AND DECREASED LIBIDO, ADULT MALE

CHIEF COMPLAINT

"Fatigue and decreased libido."

HISTORY OF PRESENT ILLNESS

A 35-year-old man with a history of HTN and obesity presents to his PCP with a complaint of fatigue. He works as an accountant and is married with three children. The patient reports that over the last year, he has gained weight, been tired, and is less motivated to work. He has also had decreased libido that is causing marital stress. He recalls that 5 years ago, he was much more active, going to the gym, and running regularly but now does not have the energy or the motivation to exercise. He has noticed a steady weight gain over the years. He has gained about 75 lbs over the last 6 years. When asked about his mood, he describes being depressed and he has not been going out with his friends or his family. He says he sometimes sleeps until someone wakes him up or he is "forced" to get up.

REVIEW OF SYSTEMS

The patient's ROS is positive for fatigue, weight gain, decreased libido, lack of motivation, and distraction at work with difficulty concentrating. His ROS is negative for dry hair or nails, constipation, palpitations, SOB, or chills.

RELEVANT HISTORY

The patient has a history is significant for HTN and obesity that developed over the last 3 years. Patient denies any surgeries and denies any family history of cancer or thyroid disease. He does report his mother has HTN. He denies drugs and tobacco. He drinks 2 to 3 beers once or twice a month.

ALLERGIES

No known drug allergies; no known food allergies.

MEDICATIONS

Lisinopril 5 mg daily.

PHYSICAL EXAMINATION

Vitals: T 36.5°C (97.8°F), R 20, P 72, BP 134/79, HT 177.8 cm (70 in.), WT 110.7 kg (244 lbs), BMI 35.

General: No acute distress, obese.

Psychiatric: Low affect.

Skin, Hair, and Nails: Normal turgor, no rash or dryness noted, no sign of hair loss.

ENT/Mouth: Moist mucosa.

Lungs: Clear to auscultation bilaterally.

Breasts: Gynecomastia bilateral, no masses.

Heart: RRR, no murmur.

Abdomen: Non-distended, non-tender, bowel sounds present.

Genital/Rectal: Testicles small bilaterally, length of testes measures approximately 3 cm bilaterally. No masses, no tenderness. No hernias. Rectal exam deferred.

Neurologic: No focal deficits.

CLINICAL DISCUSSION QUESTIONS

1. What is the differential diagnosis?

_____

_____

_____

_____

2. What is the most likely diagnosis? Why?

_____

_____

_____

_____

3. Demonstrate your understanding about the pathophysiology in regard to the most likely diagnosis.

_____

_____

_____

_____

4. Should tests/imaging studies be ordered? Which ones? Why? Think about tests/imaging beyond the primary care setting as well.

_____

_____

_____

_____

5. What are the next appropriate steps in management?

_____

_____

_____

_____

6. Review a reliable, recent source and discuss the treatment approach and contributing factors of the diagnosis. Provide references for your responses.

_____

_____

_____

_____

7. What are the pertinent ICD-10 and CPT (E/M) codes for this visit? Provide a short rationale.

_____

_____

_____

_____

8. What is the appropriate patient education for this case?

_____

_____

_____

_____

9. If not managed appropriately, what is/are the medical/legal concern(s) that may arise?

_____

_____

_____

_____

10. Think about interprofessional collaboration for this case. Provide a list of specialties or other disciplines and indicate what contribution these professionals might make to managing the patient.

_____

_____

_____

_____

BEDSIDE MANNER QUESTIONS

11. What would your communication style/approach be with this patient?

_____

_____

_____

_____

12. If a patient is distressed by the diagnosis, what might offer support?

_____

_____

_____

_____

ANSWER KEY _available at_
https://connect.springerpub.com/content/book/978-0-8261-8273-9

UNSTEADY GAIT AND NAUSEA, PEDIATRIC FEMALE

CHIEF COMPLAINT

"Unsteady gait and nausea."

HISTORY OF PRESENT ILLNESS

A 6-year-old girl is brought by her father for evaluation of an unsteady gait. Her symptoms began 3 hours ago. The child's father was initially concerned that she "might be coming down with something again" because she asked to be carried downstairs after waking up and chose to watch television before breakfast instead of playing with her siblings like she usually does. When she got up from the couch, her father noted that she walked with her feet far apart and seemed to sway to the right side. The child states her head "felt weird and heavy" when she walked, and was worse when she moved her head, "like after I spin around on my dad's office chair." Her father also states that she does not seem to be hearing well. She vomited shortly after walking back to the couch. There is no report of recent falls or injuries, and no new physical activities. The child denies headache, back pain, leg pain, and no numbness or weakness in her legs or feet. She was in the office last week and was diagnosed with a viral upper respiratory infection. The PCP recommended symptomatic treatment with nasal saline. She has been asymptomatic for the past 4 days. Currently, there no sick contacts at home or in her class at school.

REVIEW OF SYSTEMS

The child's ROS is positive for nausea, vomiting, dizziness, unsteady gait, and decreased hearing on the right. Her ROS is negative for fever, headache, cough, abdominal pain, diarrhea, constipation, eye pain, vision changes, rhinorrhea, ear pain, throat pain, upper or lower extremity pain, joint pain or swelling, numbness, or weakness.

MEDICAL HISTORY

The child had a tonsillectomy at age 5. Her immunizations are up to date including annual influenza vaccine. She lives with parents and two siblings (ages 4 and 9) with whom she plays well. She entered first grade this year and performs well in class. She has multiple friends at school. She eats three meals per day with an afternoon snack. Often, she still takes a 1-hour afternoon nap. She participates in soccer and dance classes on alternating weekends. Her parents and siblings have no significant medical history.

ALLERGIES

No known medical allergies; no known food allergies.

MEDICATIONS

None.

PHYSICAL EXAMINATION

Vitals: T 37°C (98.6°F), P 82, R 20, BP 96/58, WT 20 kg (44 lbs), HT 115 cm (45.28 in), BMI 15.1 (47th percentile).

General: Well-dressed/well-groomed, smiles, is talkative, sits very still in chair.

Skin, Hair, and Nails: Skin warm and dry, no rashes, lesions, bruising, or discoloration. No abnormal findings with hair or nails.

Head: Normocephalic, non-tender, and atraumatic.

Eyes: Pupils equal, round, and reactive to light and accommodation, extraocular eye movements intact, spontaneous left-beating horizontal nystagmus that resolves with fixation.

ENT/Mouth: Ear canal clear, tympanic membranes visible bilaterally without erythema or effusion, nares patent, turbinates pink and moist, good oral hygiene, oropharynx mucosa pink and moist.

Heart: RRR, no murmurs, brisk capillary refill, no cyanosis, distal pulses intact.

Lungs: Clear to auscultation bilaterally, chest wall movement adequate and symmetrical, no retractions or use of accessory muscles.

Abdomen: Bowel sounds active in all quadrants, soft, non-tender, non-distended.

Musculoskeletal: Ambulates without aid but waivers right when walking straight, no scoliosis or spinal abnormalities, FROM upper and lower extremities, good muscle tone, strength 5/5 upper and lower extremities.

Neurologic: A&O×3, cranial nerves II–XII grossly intact except hearing decreased on right with whisper test (VIII), DTR (patellar and Achilles tendon) 2+ bilaterally.

CLINICAL DISCUSSION QUESTIONS

1. What is the differential diagnosis?

_____

_____

_____

_____

2. What is the most likely diagnosis? Why?

_____

_____

_____

_____

3. Demonstrate your understanding about the pathophysiology in regard to the most likely diagnosis.

_____

_____

_____

_____

4. Should tests/imaging studies be ordered? Which ones? Why? Think about tests/imaging beyond the primary care setting as well.

_____

_____

_____

_____

5. What are the next appropriate steps in management?

_____

_____

_____

_____

6. What is the prevalence and what are the treatment options for this diagnosis? Provide references for your response.

_____

_____

_____

_____

7. What are the pertinent ICD-10 and CPT (E/M) codes for this visit? Provide a short rationale.

_____

_____

_____

_____

8. What are appropriate patient/parent education topics for this case?

_____

_____

_____

_____

9. If not managed appropriately, what is/are the medical/legal concern(s) that may arise?

_____

_____

_____

_____

10. Think about interprofessional collaboration for this case. Provide a list of specialties or other disciplines and indicate what contribution these professionals might make to managing the patient.

_____

_____

_____

_____

BEDSIDE MANNER QUESTION

11. What would your communication style/approach be with this patient and parent?

_____

_____

_____

_____

ANSWER KEY *available at*
https://connect.springerpub.com/content/book/978-0-8261-8273-9

EXCESS FACIAL HAIR, ADOLESCENT FEMALE

CHIEF COMPLAINT

"Excessive facial hair."

HISTORY OF PRESENT ILLNESS

An unaccompanied 16-year-old girl presents to her PCP complaining of excessive facial hair and acne. Her symptoms have increased gradually over the last 2 to 3 years along with a 60-pound weight gain since her last visit 2 years ago. The reason for this visit is she really hates the acne and dark facial hair that is causing social problems for her. She requests isotretinoin that was helpful for a friend.

The patient is less concerned about her weight but states she has tried to lose weight without success. She snacks frequently and has switched from "donuts and candy to protein bars" without success. She denies laxative use or induction of vomiting. She drinks 6 to 12 diet sodas daily. The patient is an only child and both parents often work late, leaving her frozen dinners. She avoids gym class whenever possible and does not exercise. She admits to some depressed mood and does not think fluoxetine has helped any. She takes it at her parents' request.

She denies current or past sexual activity. Menarche began age 11 with periods regular by age 12 then gradually becoming lighter and less frequent over the past 3 years. Her periods now last 2 to 3 days and occur every 6 to 8 weeks. The girl is a long-time patient of the clinic last seen 2 years ago for a well-child visit. At that time, she was diagnosed with situational (school-related) depression and acne. She was prescribed fluoxetine 20 mg daily and clindamycin 1% lotion BID. Refills are charted for the fluoxetine but not the clindamycin. Her chart contains a blanket permission from her parents to see the patient unaccompanied and she also brings a note to that effect today.

REVIEW OF SYSTEMS

The patient's ROS is positive for sleeping 9 to 10 hours most nights and some guilt about overeating sweets. Her ROS is negative for polydipsia, polyuria, polyphagia, hair loss, change in skin color or texture or thickening of facial features, tremor, palpitations, diarrhea, constipation, or suicidal or homicidal ideation.

RELEVANT HISTORY

The patient is current on all vaccinations, including HPV. She is of mixed Caucasian and African American ancestry and states other family members are not as hairy as she. She is interested in boys, but has not started dating or engaged in any romantic or sexual interaction. She denies smoking, alcohol, or drug use.

ALLERGIES

No known drug allergies; no known food allergies.

MEDICATIONS

Fluoxetine 20 mg daily for depressed mood.

PHYSICAL EXAMINATION

Vitals: T 37.1°C (98.8°F), P 80, R 14, BP 130/82, HT 165.3 cm (65 in.), WT 80.74 kg (178 lbs), BMI 29.6.

General: Talkative female in no acute distress.

Psychiatric: A&O×3 with appropriate mood and affect.

Skin, Hair, and Nails: Acne on face and upper chest and back; oily skin with papules, comedones, pustules. Mild hirsutism of face and forearms. No alopecia. No thickening or darkening of skin.

Head: Normocephalic, atraumatic.

Eyes: PERRL, EOMI.

ENT/Mouth: Nares patent, turbonates clear; TMs without erythema or effusion; dentition with multiple fillings and caries.

Chest: Symmetric excursion with no accessory muscle use.

Lungs: Resonant with vesicular breath sounds all fields, no wheezes, rales, or rhonchi.

Heart: Quiet precordium, RSR, no murmur, rub, or gallop.

Abdomen: Protuberant, normoactive bowel sounds in all quadrants, no bruit, non-tender, no masses, no costovertebral angle tenderness.

Genital/Rectal: Deferred.

Musculoskeletal: FROM and 5/5 strength in all extremities.

Neurological: Gait smooth, no tremor or past pointing.

CLINICAL DISCUSSION QUESTIONS

1. What is the differential diagnosis?

_____

_____

_____

_____

2. What is the most likely diagnosis? Why?

_____

_____

_____

_____

3. Demonstrate your understanding about the pathophysiology in regard to the most likely diagnosis.

_____

_____

_____

_____

4. Should tests/imaging studies be ordered? Which ones? Why? Think about tests/imaging beyond the primary care setting as well.

_____

_____

_____

_____

5. What are the next appropriate steps in management?

_____

_____

_____

_____

6. What is the diagnostic and management approach with this condition in adolescent patients? Provide references for your response.

_____

_____

_____

_____

7. What are the pertinent ICD-10 and CPT (E/M) codes for this visit? Provide a short rationale.

_____

_____

_____

_____

8. What is the appropriate patient education for this case?

_____

_____

_____

_____

9. If not managed appropriately, what is/are the medical/legal concern(s) that may arise?

_____

_____

_____

_____

10. Think about interprofessional collaboration for this case. Provide a list of specialties or other disciplines and indicate what contribution these professionals might make to managing the patient.

_____

_____

_____

_____

BEDSIDE MANNER QUESTION

11. What would your communication style/approach be with this patient?

_____

_____

_____

_____

ANSWER KEY *available at*
https://connect.springerpub.com/content/book/978-0-8261-8273-9

FEVER AND BODY ACHES, ADULT MALE

CHIEF COMPLAINT
"Fever and body aches."

HISTORY OF PRESENT ILLNESS
A 39-year-old male shipbuilder reports to his PCP's office in late February 2020 with a 24-hour history of fever and generalized body aches. The fever came on suddenly while he was at work yesterday and he worked through the remaining 3 hours of his shift before going home. He does not own a thermometer so did not check his temperature at home. He admits to feeling sluggish over the same period. The achiness is most pronounced in his back and shoulders and he rates it a 7/10 on a pain scale. Since onset of his symptoms, the patient admits to chills, dry cough, headache, and runny nose. He has not taken anything OTC to alleviate his symptoms. He has two children in grade school who have been sick recently but states that neither missed school because they never ran a fever. The patient is up to date on all vaccinations except annual influenza. He states that after getting the flu shot several years ago, he got the flu a few days after the vaccination and since that time has not been vaccinated.

REVIEW OF SYSTEMS
ROS is positive for generalized achiness, fever, chills, fatigue, headache, rhinorrhea, dry cough, and decrease in appetite. The patient denied ear pain, sore throat, wheezing, SOB, sinus congestion, eye pain or itching, diarrhea, nausea or vomiting, or chest pain.

RELEVANT HISTORY
The patient has a medical history of hypertension treated with lisinopril and hydrochlorothiazide. He works in a local shipyard as a welder. He is married with two children. There are no pets in the home. He does not regularly "go to the doctor" but comes to the office at least annually for his employee physical. He has smoked about 1 pack per day for the last 19 years, drinks 1 to 2 beers on the weekend, and denies the use of street drugs. His family history is unknown as he was adopted.

ALLERGIES
No known drug allergies; no known food allergies.

MEDICATIONS
Lisinopril/hydrochlorothiazide 20 mg/12.5 mg PO daily.

PHYSICAL EXAMINATION
Vitals: T 39.5°C (103.1°F), P 104, R 19, BP 130/85, HT 187.96 cm (74 in.), WT 113.85 kg (251 lbs), BMI 32.

General: Well developed, obese, in no acute distress but appears to be ill.

Psychiatric: Normal mood and affect.

ENT/Mouth: TMs pearly gray without effusion or bulging; inferior turbinates swollen, boggy, and erythematous; oropharynx without exudates but injection is present. There is no tonsillar hypertrophy. Mildly tender anterior cervical lymphadenopathy bilaterally.

Heart: Regular rhythm; mild tachycardia present; no murmurs, rubs, or gallops.

Lungs: Clear to auscultation bilaterally.

CLINICAL DISCUSSION QUESTIONS

1. What is the differential diagnosis?

_____

_____

_____

_____

2. What is the most likely diagnosis? Why?

_____

_____

_____

3. Demonstrate your understanding about the pathophysiology in regard to the most likely diagnosis.

_____

_____

_____

_____

4. Should tests/imaging studies be ordered? Which ones? Why? Think about tests/imaging beyond the primary care setting as well.

_____

_____

_____

_____

5. What are the next appropriate steps in management?

_____

_____

_____

_____

6. What are the diagnostic criteria, treatments, and prevention for this diagnosis? Provide reference/s for your responses.

_____

_____

_____

7. What are the pertinent ICD-10 and CPT (E/M) codes for this visit? Provide a short rationale.

_____

_____

_____

_____

8. What is the appropriate patient education for this case?

_____

_____

_____

_____

9. If not managed appropriately, what is/are the medical/legal concern(s) that may arise?

_____

_____

_____

_____

10. Think about interprofessional collaboration for this case. Provide a list of specialties or other disciplines and indicate what contribution these professionals might make to managing the patient.

_____

_____

_____

_____

BEDSIDE MANNER QUESTIONS

11. What would your communication style/approach be with this patient?

_____

_____

_____

_____

12. If a patient is distressed by the possibility of potentially life-threatening conditions such as COVID-19, what might offer support?

_____

_____

_____

_____

ANSWER KEY *available at*
https://connect.springerpub.com/content/book/978-0-8261-8273-9

LARGE PIMPLE ON LEG, ADULT FEMALE

CHIEF COMPLAINT

"Large pimple on leg."

HISTORY OF PRESENT ILLNESS

A 32-year-old woman presents to an urgent care clinic with a week-long history of a bump on her leg that has increased in size and pain. She wonders if she was bitten by a spider or insect and states the lesion started off about the size of a "pimple" but then kept getting larger. She was able to express some pus from it 3 to 4 days ago and thought it would go away but now it feels as if there is more tenderness underneath her skin, and although it seems to be coming a head, she cannot squeeze out any more pus. This has never happened to her before, although she does note that in the past when shaving her armpits, she sometimes would have a couple of bumps or pimples but they would usually go away after a week or two. She denies fevers, chills, or any additional systemic symptoms. She is an active athlete and goes to the gym for weight training and basketball 2 to 3 times a week and participates in a CrossFit program weekly.

REVIEW OF SYSTEMS

The patient's ROS is positive for mild fatigue and leg pain. She denies any history of abdominal pain, additional rashes or lesions, nausea/vomiting, chest pain, SOB, headache, or dizziness.

RELEVANT HISTORY

The patient's history is noncontributory. She is a cisgender heterosexual woman who reports about six sexual partners in the past 3 months. She endorses being vigilant about HIV and STI testing and endorses having negative results on HIV and all STI tests just 2 weeks ago. She works as a patient care associate at a local nursing home. The patient states she drinks at parties and social events, smokes marijuana occasionally, and reports no other drug use. Family history includes both parents with hypertension. Her only medications are daily multivitamins and oral contraceptives, and she denies any medication allergies.

ALLERGIES

No known drug allergies; no known food allergies.

MEDICATIONS

Daily multivitamins and an oral contraceptive—she did not remember the name.

PHYSICAL EXAMINATION

Vitals: T 36.8°C (98.3°F), P 88, R 12, BP 110/77, WT 68 kg (150 lbs), HT 165.1 cm (65 in.), BMI 25.

General: Well-developed, well-nourished woman in no apparent distress.

Skin, Hair, and Nails: A 3-cm nodule is noted on the right anterior thigh, with surrounding erythema and a shiny head. It is tender to palpation and there is moderate fluctuance noted as well. No other lesions or rashes are noted from a full skin exam. No abnormal findings with hair or nails.

Lungs: Clear to auscultation bilaterally.

Heart: RRR, no murmurs/rubs/gallops.

CLINICAL DISCUSSION QUESTIONS

1. What is the differential diagnosis?

_____

_____

_____

_____

2. What is the most likely diagnosis? Why?

_____

_____

_____

3. Demonstrate your understanding about the pathophysiology in regard to the most likely diagnosis.

_____

_____

_____

_____

4. Should tests/imaging studies be ordered? Which ones? Why? Think about tests/imaging beyond the primary care setting as well.

_____

_____

_____

_____

5. What are the next appropriate steps in management?

_____

_____

_____

6. What are the treatment options and the recurrence of the diagnosis? Provide references for your response.

_____

_____

_____

7. What are the pertinent ICD-10 and CPT (E/M) codes for this visit? Provide a short rationale.

_____

_____

8. What is the appropriate patient education for this case?

_____

_____

_____

_____

9. If not managed appropriately, what is/are the medical/legal concern(s) that may arise?

_____

_____

_____

_____

10. Think about interprofessional collaboration for this case. Provide a list of specialties or other disciplines and indicate what contribution these professionals might make to managing the patient.

_____

_____

_____

_____

BEDSIDE MANNER QUESTION

11. What would your communication style/approach be with this patient?

_____

_____

_____

_____

ANSWER KEY *available at*
https://connect.springerpub.com/content/book/978-0-8261-8273-9

CHEST PAIN, ADULT FEMALE

CHIEF COMPLAINT
"Chest pain."

HISTORY OF PRESENT ILLNESS
A 28-year-old Caucasian woman who is a military spouse presents after a visit to an ED for recurrent episodes of chest pain. Approximately 1 year ago, she began waking abruptly at night feeling "like I'm going to die," with trembling, SOB, racing pulse, and chest discomfort, lasting for 10 to 15 minutes. Her chest discomfort is described as diffuse tightness, without radiation, sweating, or nausea. Episodes were somewhat relieved by getting out of bed, walking around, and opening a window for fresh air. These episodes occurred every 3 to 4 weeks, with no known triggers; they were becoming frequent and disabling as she anticipated a recurrence. In recent months, her distress had resulted in three visits to the local ED, where she was evaluated for cardiac and pulmonary disease, ruling out AMI, angina, pulmonary embolus, and hypoglycemia (EKG, cardiac enzymes, blood work, chest X-ray were all normal). She was told "It's in your head" and not to worry about a heart attack.

The patient's main concern was that she would keep having these frightening episodes and that medical professionals could not help.

REVIEW OF SYSTEMS
The patient's ROS is positive for loneliness and anxiety that began when her husband was deployed to the Middle East. Other psychiatric symptoms are negative: depression, suicidal ideation, memory problems. Her ROS is negative for fever, night sweats, weight loss, loss of appetite, loss of energy, loss of concentration, lack or excessive sleep, loss of interest, skipped heart beats, extremity swelling, wheezing, cough, nocturia/orthopnea, and heartburn.

MEDICAL HISTORY
The patient's history is negative for major illnesses or injuries. She denies psychologic or emotional trauma. Her last routine health maintenance exam was 11 months ago for well-woman visit; results were normal.

Her immunizations are up to date. She is married to an army infantry soldier who is deployed to the Middle East. They have been married 3 years and have no children. Her family lives in a different state. She denies alcohol, tobacco, or recreational drug use. She regularly walks 2 miles for exercise.

ALLERGIES
No known drug allergies; no known food allergies.

MEDICATION
Levonorgestrel IUD ×3 years.

PHYSICAL EXAMINATION

Vitals: T 37°C (98.7°F), P 80, R 14, BP 124/80 mmHg, HT 165 cm (65 in.), WT 62.5 kg (138 lbs), BMI 23, pulse ox 99%.

General: Well-developed, well-nourished woman appearing stated age.

Psychiatric: A&O×3, anxious appearance.

Neck: No thyromegaly, nodules, bruits, or adenopathy.

ENT/Mouth: Posterior pharynx unobstructed.

Heart: RRR; no murmurs, gallops, rubs, clicks; PMI non-displaced.

Lungs: Clear to auscultation bilaterally; no wheezes, rales, rhonchi, symmetric expansion; no chest wall tenderness.

Abdomen: BS all quadrants, soft, non-tender; no hepatosplenomegaly, no masses.

Extremities: Pulses 2+ and equal; no tenderness, redness, swelling, or varicosities.

CLINICAL DISCUSSION QUESTIONS

1. What is the differential diagnosis?

_____

_____

_____

_____

2. What is the most likely diagnosis? Why?

_____

_____

_____

_____

3. Demonstrate your understanding about the pathophysiology in regard to the most likely diagnosis.

_____

_____

_____

_____

4. Should tests/imaging studies be ordered? Which ones? Why? Think about tests/imaging beyond the primary care setting as well.

_____

_____

_____

_____

5. What are the next appropriate steps in management?

_____

_____

_____

_____

6. Review recent and credible research articles about this diagnosis. Demonstrate your understanding of the prevalence specific to this patient type and treatment options for the diagnosis. Provide references.

_____

_____

_____

_____

7. What are the pertinent ICD-10 and CPT (E/M) codes for this visit? Provide a short rationale.

_____

_____

_____

_____

8. What is the appropriate patient education for this case?

_____

_____

_____

_____

9. If not managed appropriately, what is/are the medical/legal concern(s) that may arise?

_____

_____

_____

_____

10. Think about interprofessional collaboration for this case. Provide a list of specialties or other disciplines and indicate what contribution these professionals might make to managing the patient.

_____

_____

_____

_____

BEDSIDE MANNER QUESTIONS

11. What would your communication style/approach be with this patient?

_____

_____

_____

_____

12. If a patient was unsure if the treatment plan is effective, how would you handle her concern?

_____

_____

_____

_____

ANSWER KEY _available at_
https://connect.springerpub.com/content/book/978-0-8261-8273-9

RIGHT KNEE PAIN, GERIATRIC MALE

CHIEF COMPLAINT

"Right knee pain."

HISTORY OF PRESENT ILLNESS

A 65-year-old man with a history of hypertension and dyslipidemia presents with right knee pain. This is his first visit to the clinic. The patient states the knee has been painful for 6 months and is exacerbated by prolonged standing and walking, pivoting, and going from sitting to standing. He also complains of start-up pain and pain at night. The patient denies any knee snapping but does complain of an occasional audible grinding sensation in the right knee.

The patient has tried massage therapy and ibuprofen with little to no benefit. He rates his pain is 10 of 10 today and 7 of 10 on most days. The patient complains of occasional popping and locking of the knee but no giving-away symptoms. The patient is community ambulatory but uses a three-prong cane due to his pain.

REVIEW OF SYSTEMS

The patient's ROS is negative for fever, chills, vomiting, diarrhea, constipation, SOB, and chest pain. He denies any altered sensation or weakness of both extremities, any temperature changes to the feet, any recent illnesses or hospitalizations, and any radicular pain or paresthesia.

RELEVANT HISTORY

The patient has a history of controlled hypertension and dyslipidemia. He uses CBD oil, drinks occasionally, and does not smoke. His family history is noncontributory.

ALLERGIES

- No known drug allergies.
- No known food allergies.

MEDICATIONS

- Lisinopril 40 mg 1 tablet PO QD
- Lovastatin 20 mg 1 tablet PO QD
- Ibuprofen 200 mg PRN for pain

PHYSICAL EXAMINATION

Vitals: T 6.5°C (97.7°F), P 64, R 20, BP 134/88, WT 142 kg (313 lbs), HT 177.8 cm (70 in.), BMI 45.

General: Morbidly obese male in no apparent distress.

Musculoskeletal: Right knee range of motion is expressed in degrees; range of motion, actual/normal—extension: 0/0; flexion: 130/130. Mild effusion. No skin lesions or abrasions. While standing, the patient has excessive varus alignment, which is not present on the contralateral leg. There is no patellofemoral crepitus or patellar instability. The patella tracks well clinically. There is no tenderness around the patellofemoral joint. Patellofemoral compression test is negative. The Q-angle is normal. There is no tenderness in the medial parapatellar region or painful medial patellar cord. The patient has no instability to varus/valgus test in full extension, 30° or 90° of flexion. Testing for anterior cruciate ligament instability produced negative results for Lachman, anterior drawer, and pivot shift tests. Testing for posterior cruciate ligament instability is negative. Quadricep strength is 5/5. Tenderness over the medial joint line and positive McMurray test when loading the medial compartment. The compression/rotation test is positive. There is no tenderness over the medial proximal tibia (below the joint line). The patient has full extension against resistance without difficulty. There are good pulses distally.

Neurologic: Sensation intact to the dorsal and plantar aspects of the foot, ankle, and leg. No signs of foot drop. No altered sensation compared to the contralateral extremity. No ankle clonus. Achilles reflex 2+.

CLINICAL DISCUSSION QUESTIONS

1. What is the differential diagnosis?

_____

_____

_____

2. What is the most likely diagnosis? Why?

_____

_____

_____

3. Demonstrate your understanding about the pathophysiology in regard to the most likely diagnosis.

_____

_____

_____

4. Should tests/imaging studies be ordered? Which ones? Why? Think about tests/imaging beyond the primary care setting as well.

_____

_____

_____

5. What are the next appropriate steps in management?

_____

_____

_____

6. Review a recent and credible research article(s) about this diagnosis. Demonstrate your understanding of the diagnostic criteria, treatment options, and risk factors of the diagnosis. Include your reference(s).

_____

_____

_____

_____

7. What are the pertinent ICD-10 and CPT (E/M) codes for this visit? Provide a short rationale.

_____

_____

_____

8. What is the appropriate patient education for this case?

_____

_____

_____

_____

9. If not managed appropriately, what is/are the medical/legal concern(s) that may arise?

_____

_____

_____

_____

10. Think about interprofessional collaboration for this case. Provide a list of specialties or other disciplines and indicate what contribution these professionals might make to managing the patient.

_____

_____

_____

_____

BEDSIDE MANNER QUESTION
11. What would your communication style/approach be with this patient?

_____

_____

_____

_____

ANSWER KEY _available at_
https://connect.springerpub.com/content/book/978-0-8261-8273-9

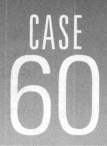

PAINFUL URINATION, ADOLESCENT MALE

CHIEF COMPLAINT
"Burning sensation while urinating."

HISTORY OF PRESENT ILLNESS
A 17-year-old male with no significant medical history presents with a complaint of urinary symptoms. He reports that for the last week, he has noticed mild burning with urination. He has noticed a thick and white/yellow penile discharge. He states he had unprotected sex with a new partner about 2 weeks ago. His partner is asymptomatic. He has not been tested for STIs in the past. He has had four sexual partners in the last 2 years and claims his last sexual encounter was unprotected. He has had unprotected sex in the past. He has noticed slight testicular discomfort, with 2/10 pain. He is concerned about these symptoms and asking about what he could have. He denies fever and genital lesions.

REVIEW OF SYSTEMS
The patient's ROS is positive for dysuria, penile discharge, and testicular pain. The ROS is negative for fever, recent illnesses, chest pain, SOB, abdominal pain, diarrhea, constipation, nausea, vomiting, and mood change.

RELEVANT HISTORY
The patient is a senior in high school with no known medical problems or surgical history. His immunizations are up to date. He denies regular tobacco use but has vaped a few times. He drinks alcohol at parties maybe once every 1 to 2 months. He experimented with marijuana once but denies other illicit drug usage. He works at a department store at the local mall.

ALLERGIES
No known drug allergies; no known food allergies.

MEDICATIONS
None.

PHYSICAL EXAMINATION
Vitals: T 36.5°C (97.8°F), P 103, R 20, BP 115/78, HT 172.7 cm (68 in.), WT 71.7 kg (158 lbs), BMI 24.

General: No acute distress.

Psychiatric: Normal affect. Responds to questions appropriately.

Skin, Hair, and Nails: No rashes or skin lesions visible. No abnormal findings with hair or nails.

Head: Normocephalic, atraumatic.

Chest: No labored breathing, chest symmetrical.

Lungs: Clear to auscultation bilaterally; no wheezing, rhonchi, or rales.

Heart: Mild tachycardia, no murmur appreciated.

Abdomen: Non-tender, non-distended, normal bowel sound.

Genital/Rectal: Uncircumcised penis, no skin lesions. Mild tenderness to epididymis on right side, scant white discharge from urethra.

Neurologic: No focal deficits.

CLINICAL DISCUSSION QUESTIONS

1. What is the differential diagnosis?

_____

_____

_____

_____

2. What is the most likely diagnosis? Why?

_____

_____

_____

_____

3. Demonstrate your understanding about the pathophysiology in regard to the most likely diagnosis.

_____

_____

_____

_____

4. Should tests/imaging studies be ordered? Which ones? Why? Think about tests/imaging beyond the primary care setting as well.

_____

_____

_____

_____

5. What are the next appropriate steps in management?

_____

_____

_____

_____

6. What are the incidence, treatment options, and treatment approach for this diagnosis? Provide references for your response.

_____

_____

_____

7. What are the pertinent ICD-10 and CPT (C/M) codes for this visit? Provide a short rationale.

---

8. What is the appropriate patient education for this case?

---

9. If not managed appropriately, what is/are the medical/legal concern(s) that may arise?

---

10. Think about interprofessional collaboration for this case. Provide a list of specialties or other disciplines and indicate what contribution these professionals might make to managing the patient.

BEDSIDE MANNER QUESTION
11. What would your communication style/approach be with this patient?

PERSISTENT BAD COUGH, ADULT FEMALE

CHIEF COMPLAINT

"Persistent bad cough."

HISTORY OF PRESENT ILLNESS

A 50-year-old woman presents to her PCP with a complaint of ongoing dry, non-productive cough for 4 weeks with intermittent harsh coughing episodes, burning chest, and SOB. She states she had an upper respiratory infection 4 weeks ago that resolved after 2 weeks. She states the cough lingered and worsened. There is an increase in mucous, and SOB has developed. The cough is worse at night or when talking. She is having difficulty doing her job, where she is expected to talk for long periods. For the last week, she has been taking frequent puffs of an albuterol rescue inhaler she has for asthma. She states she is fatigued and thinks she is getting worse. Her family complains of the frequent loud and harsh cough. She thinks the recent forest fires and bad air quality in her area have contributed to her cough. She states most of the family who lives with her also developed a "cold" around the same time, but they are all doing well now, except her.

REVIEW OF SYSTEMS

The patient's ROS is positive for a harsh, frequent, non-productive cough with intermittent SOB. She denies a history of smoking cigarettes or other inhalants but states she grew up with parents who smoked in the home. She had a flu shot 6 weeks ago. Her ROS is negative for fever, hemoptysis, wheezing, chest pain, night sweats, poor appetite, body aches, pain, ear pain, nasal congestion, sore throat, history of pneumonia or lung disease, nausea, vomiting, diarrhea, recent travel, exposure to tuberculosis, or rash. She states her asthma and acid reflux are controlled with routine medication.

RELEVANT HISTORY

The patient's history is relevant for seasonal allergies, asthma, and acid reflux disease. Surgical history includes tonsillectomy and adenoidectomy (age 14). She is up to date on immunizations. She is a full-time high school teacher. She denies smoking and recreational drug use but does enjoy one drink, usually wine, several days per week. Her exercise level is usually light to moderate but since getting sick she has been sedentary. Her family history is significant for asthma and seasonal allergies.

ALLERGIES

No known drug allergies; no known food allergies.

MEDICATIONS

- Fluticasone propionate/salmeterol inhaled 250/50, 1 puff BID.
- Albuterol rescue inhaler, q4-6h PRN.
- Esomeprazole, 40 mg PO QD.
- Fluticasone propionate nasal spray, 1 spray in each nostril PRN.

PHYSICAL EXAMINATION

Vitals: T 36.9°C (98.4°F), P 100, R 20, BP 126/82, SpO_2 96%, HT 162.56 cm (64 in.), WT 74.4 kg (164 lbs), BMI 28.

General: Well dressed with good hygiene. Appears tired.

Psychiatric: Cooperative with exam and appropriate to situation.

Skin, Hair, and Nails: No rash. No abnormal findings with hair or nails.

Eyes: PERRL, sclera clear.

ENT/Mouth: TMs present bilaterally with good light reflex. No tenderness to palpation. Nares patent and pale and body with small amount clear drainage. Oral mucosa moist and normal. Normal dentation. Pharynx normal.

Neck: No cervical or pre- or post-auricular lymphadenopathy. No tenderness. FROM.

Chest: Symmetrical.

Lungs: Positive for frequent, dry, and loud cough, non-productive. Coughing increases with talking and deep breaths. Lungs were mostly clear with a scattered wheeze bilaterally. No rhonchi or crackles.

Heart: RRR. No murmur.

Abdomen: BS present. Abdomen soft with no tenderness to palpation.

Neurologic: A&O×3.

CLINICAL DISCUSSION QUESTIONS

1. What is the differential diagnosis?

_____

_____

_____

_____

2. What is the most likely diagnosis? Why?

_____

_____

_____

_____

3. Demonstrate your understanding about the pathophysiology in regard to the most likely diagnosis.

_____

_____

_____

_____

_____

4. Should tests/imaging studies be ordered? Which ones? Why? Think about tests/imaging beyond the primary care setting as well.

_____

_____

_____

_____

_____

5. What are the next appropriate steps in management?

_____

_____

_____

_____

_____

6. Review a reliable, recent reference and demonstrate an understanding of prescribing antibiotics for this diagnosis. Include the references.

_____

_____

_____

_____

_____

7. What are the pertinent ICD-10 and CPT (E/M) codes for this visit? Provide a short rationale.

_____

_____

_____

_____

8. What are appropriate patient education topics for this case?

_____

_____

_____

_____

_____

9. If not managed appropriately, what is/are the medical/legal concern(s) that may arise?

_____

_____

_____

_____

_____

10. Think about interprofessional collaboration for this case. Provide a list of specialties or other disciplines and indicate what contribution these professionals might make to managing the patient.

_____

_____

_____

_____

_____

BEDSIDE MANNER QUESTION
11. What would your communication style/approach be with this patient?

_____

_____

_____

_____

ANSWER KEY _available at_
https://connect.springerpub.com/content/book/978-0-8261-8273-9

ADULT WELL VISIT, GERIATRIC MALE

CHIEF COMPLAINT

"Adult well visit."

HISTORY OF PRESENT ILLNESS

A 66-year-old man presents to his PCP for his annual adult well visit and a 6-month history of fatigue that he attributes to waking up 2 to 3 times a night to urinate. He is not too concerned because some of his friends experience similar symptoms. There have been no dietary, social, or environmental changes in his life during the past year. He is not taking any prescription or over-the-counter medications. He states he generally feels well, exercises 3 times a week for 30 minutes a day, eats healthy organic foods as much as possible. He has no chronic illnesses or relevant medical history.

REVIEW OF SYSTEMS

The patient's ROS is positive for mild fatigue, sleep disturbance, nocturia, decreased urinary stream, some urinary hesitancy, and occasional dribbling. His ROS is negative for fever, unexplained weight loss, SOB, polyuria, polydipsia, dysuria, hematuria, urethral discharge, urinary urgency, urinary frequency, and incontinence.

RELEVANT HISTORY

The patient's history is negative for major illnesses and trauma. As part of a comprehensive annual visit, a review of his last routine lab tests, colonoscopy, vision, and hearing tests are negative. His immunizations are up to date including tetanus, diphtheria, acellular pertussis, pneumococcal 13-valent conjugate (1 year ago), recombinant zoster, and influenza vaccines.

His social history includes drinking 1 to 2 beers per week since age 20 and an average of 3 cups of coffee per day. The patient has been a bodybuilder since his 30s, working out with weights 3 times a week. He and his husband walk 2 miles together on most mornings. HIV risk factors were assessed. The patient has one sex partner (husband) and engages in both insertive and receptive anal sex 2 to 3 times a week. His partner has no other sexual partners. A screen for STIs prior to their marriage 10 years ago was negative for gonorrhea, chlamydia, syphilis, hepatitis B, hepatitis C, and HIV. His family history is significant in that his father died of prostate cancer at 68 years of age. He has no uncles or brothers.

ALLERGIES

No known drug allergies; no known food allergies.

MEDICATIONS

None.

PHYSICAL EXAMINATION

Vitals: T 37.0°C (98.6°F), P 76, R 14, BP 122/80 mm Hg, HT 183 cm (72 in.), WT 82 kg (180.8 lbs), BMI 24.5.

General: Well-developed, well-nourished male in no acute distress.

Psychiatric: Appears slightly anxious and somewhat fatigued.

Skin, Hair, and Nails: No rashes or lesions. Hair and nails with no abnormal findings.

Eyes: Vision 20/20 with corrective lenses on Snellen test.

ENT/Mouth: Hearing grossly intact.

Neck: Thyroid not enlarged, no palpable nodules.

Chest: Chest expansion is symmetrical.

Heart: RRR without murmur or gallop.

Lungs: Clear to auscultation bilaterally.

Abdomen: Active bowel sounds; abdomen soft, non-tender; no masses.

Genital/Rectal: Uncircumcised male, no discharge or lesions, no scrotal or testicular masses. Soft, non-tender, symmetrical, boggy, 2+ enlarged prostate, loss of median sulcus; no palpable prostate nodules.

Musculoskeletal: No tenderness; full range of motion on BUE and BLE.

Neurologic: A&O, cranial nerves II to XII intact.

CLINICAL DISCUSSION QUESTIONS

1. What is the differential diagnosis?

2. What is the most likely diagnosis? Why?

3. Demonstrate your understanding about the pathophysiology in regard to the most likely diagnosis.

4. Should tests/imaging studies be ordered? Which ones? Why? Think about tests/imaging beyond the primary care setting as well.

5. What are the next appropriate steps in management?

    _____
    _____
    _____
    _____
    _____

6. Discuss severity of symptoms, initial preferred treatment, how treatment can affect sexual function, and activities that can affect relevant blood tests for this diagnosis. Provide references to support your statements.

    _____
    _____
    _____
    _____
    _____

7. What are the pertinent ICD-10 and CPT (E/M) codes for this visit? Provide a short rationale.

    _____
    _____
    _____
    _____
    _____

8. What is the appropriate patient education for this case?

    _____
    _____
    _____
    _____

9. If not managed appropriately, what is/are the medical/legal concern(s) that may arise?

    _____
    _____
    _____
    _____

10. Think about interprofessional collaboration for this case. Provide a list of specialties or other disciplines and indicate what contribution these professionals might make to managing the patient.

_____

_____

_____

_____

_____

BEDSIDE MANNER QUESTIONS

11. What would your communication style/approach be with this patient?

_____

_____

_____

_____

_____

12. If a patient is distressed by the diagnosis, what might offer support?

_____

_____

_____

_____

_____

ANSWER KEY *available at*
https://connect.springerpub.com/content/book/978-0-8261-8273-9

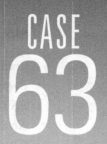

LOW PLATELETS, ADULT MALE

CHIEF COMPLAINT
"Low platelets."

HISTORY OF PRESENT ILLNESS
A new patient, age 42, is referred by his health insurance helpline to establish care and to discuss "low platelets" noted on a recent life insurance blood test. He has been without a PCP since college and has no prior labs for comparison. He feels completely well, stating he rarely gets sick, using the local urgent care center rarely for colds and minor injuries. He denies any unusual bleeding, bruising, or skin changes. There is no known personal or family history of blood or liver disorders.

REVIEW OF SYSTEMS
The patient's ROS is negative for fever, chills, weight loss, or fatigue. He has no nasal congestion, earache, or sore throat. He reports no vision changes, tearing, or redness/yellowing of the eyes; no cough, SOB, or wheezing; no chest pain, palpitations, or edema; no abdominal pain, nausea, vomiting, reflux, melena, change in bowel movements, or rectal bleeding; no rashes, jaundice, pruritus, or skin lesions; no bruising, epistaxis, or swollen lymph nodes; no headache, dizziness, weakness, or paresthesia; no insomnia, depression, or anxiety.

RELEVANT HISTORY
The patient underwent an appendectomy as a child but has no other hospitalizations or medical diagnoses. He denies taking any prescription or OTC medications, herbs, vitamins, or other supplements. He had all childhood vaccines and receives annual flu shots from an urgent care clinic. His family history is significant for diabetes (mother and brother). The patient is married and has two young children. He is the director of sales for a local winery, working 50 hours per week; and has worked there for 17 years. He drinks 3 to 4 glasses of wine daily, which he describes as a "necessary part of my job." He has never had any work, home, or legal problems related to alcohol, and he denies binges, cravings, or withdrawal symptoms. He has never used tobacco or recreational drugs. He eats out 4 days per week: steak, potatoes, pasta, bread; his wife cooks his favorite foods at home, including carne asada with tortillas, rice, and beans. His exercise is limited to taking his kids to a park once a week.

ALLERGIES
None.

MEDICATIONS
None.

PHYSICAL EXAMINATION
Vitals: T 36.9°C (98.4°F), P 82, R 16, BP 138/84, SpO$_2$ 99%, HT 175.26 cm (69 in.), WT 108.9 kg (240 lbs), BMI 35.

General: Well-developed, over-nourished Latinx, A&O×3, all vital signs stable. In no acute distress.

Psychiatric: Pleasant affect, euthymic mood, fluent speech, good insight.

Skin, Hair, and Nails: Skin warm and dry. Moderate palmar erythema present bilaterally. Two small spider angiomas of anterior chest but no jaundice, rashes, or varicosities noted. No abnormal findings with hair and nail exam.

Eyes: PERRLA, conjunctivae clear, no scleral icterus.

ENT/Mouth: No oropharyngeal lesions.

Neck: Supple with no lymphadenopathy or thyromegaly.

Chest: No gynecomastia or axillary lymphadenopathy noted.

Heart: RRR with no murmurs, gallops, or rubs. Carotid and radial pulses are 2+ bilaterally.

Lungs: Lungs clear to auscultation with no adventitious sounds noted.

Abdomen: Protuberant with central adiposity and well-healed surgical scar at RLQ; no caput medusae, bulging flanks, or fluid wave present. Normal active bowel sounds noted in all quadrants with no bruits or friction rubs. Normal areas of tympany and dullness to percussion noted. Soft, non-tender; no masses or hernia appreciated. Hepatomegaly with liver span percussing to 20 cm at the mid-clavicular line; palpated liver edge is firm but smooth and non-tender. Spleen tip is palpable but non-tender.

Musculoskeletal: No muscle atrophy; trace pitting edema of bilateral pretibial areas; no presacral edema, clubbing, or cyanosis.

Neurologic: Normal gait; no tremors or asterixis present; no focal deficits noted.

Diagnostic Tests: Labs brought in by patient dated 1 month prior to visit:

- WBC = 8.9×10^3/uL
- Hgb = 15.0 g/dL
- Hct = 44.1%
- MCV = 99 fL (H)
- Platelets = 112×10^3/uL (L)
- Peripheral smear = Platelet numbers low; no clumping or giant forms; mormal lymphocyte morphology
- BUN = 16 mg/dL
- Creatinine = 1.00 mg/dL
- Sodium = 136 mmol/L
- Chloride = 102 mmol/L
- Potassium = 4.8 mmol/L
- Calcium = 9.9 mg/dL
- Glucose = 100 mg/dL (H)
- Albumin = 3.6 g/dL (L)
- Protein = 6.2 g/dL
- ALT = 28 IU/L
- AST = 40 IU/L
- ALP = 141 IU/L
- Tbili = 1.2 mg/dL
- Dbili = 0.8 mg/dL (H)
- HbA1C = 6.0 (H)
- HCVAb = negative
- HBsAb = positive
- HBcAb = neg
- HBsAg = neg
- HIV Ab = neg
- Total cholesterol = 212 mg/dL (H)
- HDL = 39 mg/dL (L)
- LDL = 142 mg/dL (H)
- Trigs = 386 mg/dL (H)

CLINICAL DISCUSSION QUESTIONS

1. What is the differential diagnosis?

_____

_____

_____

_____

2. What is the most likely diagnosis? Why?

_____

_____

_____

_____

3. Demonstrate your understanding about the pathophysiology in regard to the most likely diagnosis.

_____

_____

_____

_____

4. Should tests/imaging studies be ordered? Which ones? Why? Think about tests/imaging beyond the primary care setting as well.

_____

_____

_____

_____

5. What are the next appropriate steps in management?

_____

_____

_____

_____

6. Demonstrate your understanding of the prevalence, screening for early intervention, and prognosis associated with the condition. Provide references to your response.

_____

_____

_____

_____

7. What are the pertinent ICD-10 and CPT (E/M) codes for this visit? Provide a short rationale.

_____

_____

_____

_____

8. What is the appropriate patient education for this case?

_____

_____

_____

_____

9. If not managed appropriately, what is/are the medical/legal concern(s) that may arise?

_____

_____

_____

_____

10. Think about interprofessional collaboration for this case. Provide a list of specialties or other disciplines and indicate what contribution these professionals might make to managing the patient.

_____

_____

_____

_____

BEDSIDE MANNER QUESTIONS

11. What would your communication style/approach be with this patient?

_____

_____

_____

_____

_____

12. If the patient is distressed by the diagnosis, what might offer support?

_____

_____

_____

_____

_____

ANSWER KEY _available at_
https://connect.springerpub.com/content/book/978-0-8261-8273-9

SKIN LESIONS AFTER SUN EXPOSURE, ADULT FEMALE

CHIEF COMPLAINT

"Skin lesions after sun exposure."

HISTORY OF PRESENT ILLNESS

A 39-year-old woman presents to her PCP for an evaluation of a rash and lesions on her face and neck that she states become worse with sun exposure. These lesions began about 12 weeks ago. She recently saw a dermatologist, who suggested she may have lupus and needed further workup for definitive diagnosis. She has returned to her PCP for a second opinion. The patient reports these lesions are itchy and at times painful, and they seem to heal in a few days. She also complains of moderate fatigue in the past 6 weeks but is otherwise a healthy female.

REVIEW OF SYSTEMS

The patient's ROS is positive for photosensitivity, rash on face and neck for 12 weeks, and fatigue for 6 weeks. Her ROS is negative for headache, nausea, dyspepsia, weight loss, unexplained fever, adenopathy, oral ulcers, arthralgia, myalgia, edema, or anxiety. She denies moles of changing color.

RELEVANT HISTORY

The patient has a history of obesity, prediabetes, and hypertension. She is up to date on vaccines, Pap smears, and dental visits.

ALLERGIES

No known drug allergies; no known food allergies.

MEDICATIONS

Hydrochlorothiazide/lisinopril 12.5 mg/10 mg QD.

PHYSICAL EXAMINATION

Vitals: T 36.6°C (97.8°F), P 82, R 18, BP 143/84, HT 167.6 cm (66 in.), WT 95.7 kg (211 lbs), BMI 34.1.

General: No acute distress.

Psychiatric: Mildly anxious.

Skin, Hair, and Nails: Multiple erythematous patches and plaques with scaling noted on face and both hands. No abnormal findings with hair or nails.

ENT/Mouth: TMs clear, no lesion or ulcers noted inside oropharyngeal mucosa.

Neck: Supple, no lymphadenopathy noted.

Lungs: Clear to auscultation bilaterally with symmetrical chest expansion.

Heart: RRR, no murmur or gallops heard.

Musculoskeletal: ROM within normal limit both bilateral upper and lower extremity.

Neurologic: A&O×3, no focal deficits noted on exam.

CLINICAL DISCUSSION QUESTIONS

1. What is the differential diagnosis?

_____

_____

_____

_____

2. What is the most likely diagnosis? Why?

_____

_____

_____

_____

3. Demonstrate your understanding about the pathophysiology in regard to the most likely diagnosis.

_____

_____

_____

_____

4. Should tests/imaging studies be ordered? Which ones? Why? Think about tests/imaging beyond the primary care setting as well.

_____

_____

_____

_____

5. What are the next appropriate steps in management?

_____

_____

_____

_____

6. What are the risk factors and treatment options for this diagnosis? Provide references for your responses.

_____

_____

_____

_____

7. What are the pertinent ICD-10 and CPT (E/M) codes for this visit? Provide a short rationale.

_____

_____

_____

_____

8. What is the appropriate patient education for this case?

_____

_____

_____

_____

9. If not managed appropriately, what is/are the medical/legal concern(s) that may arise?

_____

_____

_____

_____

10. Think about interprofessional collaboration for this case. Provide a list of specialties or other disciplines and indicate what contribution these professionals might make to managing the patient.

_____

_____

_____

_____

_____

BEDSIDE MANNER QUESTION
11. What would your communication style/approach be with this patient?

_____

_____

_____

_____

_____

ANSWER KEY *available at*
https://connect.springerpub.com/content/book/978-0-8261-8273-9

DAYTIME FATIGUE, ADULT MALE

CHIEF COMPLAINT
"Daytime fatigue."

HISTORY OF PRESENT ILLNESS
A 46-year-old man with a medical history of essential hypertension presents to his PCP for an evaluation of excessive daytime sleepiness and generalized fatigue. He works a 5-day week as an accountant and often works an extra Saturday or two each month. The patient states he often yawns throughout the day and at times has taken naps during the workday. There have been occasions when coworkers have had to wake him at his desk. The patient is accompanied by his wife, who has been increasingly concerned that her husband wakes up multiple times throughout the night with a choking sensation. This has been ongoing for the past several months but has increased in frequency. She also noticed he often gasps for air each time he wakes up with this choking sensation. When asked about snoring, the patient denies he snores, but the wife states he has always snored very loud, especially over the past year and a half. There are times his wife thinks he stops breathing at night. He has never been hospitalized and he is adherent with his antihypertensive medications. The patient seldom exercises.

REVIEW OF SYSTEMS
The patient's ROS is positive for occasional palpitations, weight gain (30 lbs), anxiety, and insomnia. The ROS is negative for fever, chills, headaches, visual disturbances, sore throat, SOB, chest pain, abdomen pain, sudden loss of muscle tone, sleep paralysis, nausea/vomiting, focal numbness or weakness, tingling, increased hunger or thirst, hallucinations, poor concentration, lack of appetite, sadness, and suicidal thoughts.

RELEVANT HISTORY
The patient's history is significant for essential hypertension diagnosed at age 36, and he has no history of drug, tobacco, or alcohol use. He reports a family history of hypertension and obesity. The patient lives at home with his wife, they have been married for 5 years, and he describes his marriage and family life as happy and healthy. They have two children.

ALLERGIES
No known drug allergies; no known food allergies.

MEDICATIONS
Amlodipine 5 mg PO daily.

PHYSICAL EXAMINATION
Vitals: T 36.8°C (98.2°F), P 88, R 18, BP 140/85, WT 102.05 kg (225 lbs), HT 172.72 cm (68 in.), BMI 34.2.

General: No apparent distress, appears stated age.

Psychiatric: Normal affect, no disorganized behavior.

Skin, Hair, and Nails: No rashes, normal skin turgor, normal hair texture, nails without splinter hemorrhages or clubbing.

Head: Normocephalic, atraumatic, no lesions.

Eyes: PERRL, anicteric sclerae.

ENT/Mouth: Mucous membranes moist, no oral cavity lesions, oropharynx without erythema.

Neck: Large neck circumference 18 in. (45.7 cm), no thyromegaly.

Chest: No obvious pectus deformity, normal excursion.

Lungs: Unlabored respirations, clear to auscultation bilaterally.

Heart: RRR, no murmurs, S1 and S2 present with normal timing.

Abdomen: No striae, soft, non-tender; bowel sounds are present and normoactive; waist circumference is 44 in. (111.7 cm).

Musculoskeletal: Symmetric distribution of muscle bulk throughout; no point tenderness along spinal column.

Neurologic: A&O×3, cranial nerves II to XII intact, motor strength is 5/5 at the upper extremity and lower extremity bilaterally; no gross sensory deficits.

CLINICAL DISCUSSION QUESTIONS

1. What is the differential diagnosis?

_____

_____

_____

_____

2. What is the most likely diagnosis? Why?

_____

_____

_____

_____

3. Demonstrate your understanding about the pathophysiology in regard to the most likely diagnosis.

_____

_____

_____

_____

4. Should tests/imaging studies be ordered? Which ones? Why? Think about tests/imaging beyond the primary care setting as well.

_____

_____

_____

_____

5. What are the next appropriate steps in management?

_____

_____

_____

_____

6. What are the screening methods and diagnostic approaches for this diagnosis? Provide reference(s) to your response.

_____

_____

_____

_____

7. What are the pertinent ICD-10 and CPT (E/M) codes for this visit? Provide a short rationale.

_____

_____

_____

_____

8. What is the appropriate patient education for this case?

_____

_____

_____

_____

9. If not managed appropriately, what is/are the medical/legal concern(s) that may arise?

_____

_____

_____

_____

10. Think about interprofessional collaboration for this case. Provide a list of specialties or other disciplines and indicate what contribution these professionals might make to managing the patient.

_____

_____

_____

_____

BEDSIDE MANNER QUESTION

11. What would your communication style/approach be with this patient?

_____

_____

_____

_____

ANSWER KEY *available at*
https://connect.springerpub.com/content/book/978-0-8261-8273-9

SHORTNESS OF BREATH, GERIATRIC MALE

CHIEF COMPLAINT

"Shortness of breath."

HISTORY OF PRESENT ILLNESS

A 74-year-old man presents for SOB, cough, wheezing, and fatigue for 1 week. His SOB and cough have worsened in the past 3 days, prompting him to seek care at the clinic. He denies fever, sweating, or chills. The patient states that he has been getting "winded" when he walks to his mailbox (approximately 60 ft.). On further questioning, the patient admits to smoking one pack of cigarettes a day for the past 50 years and has no desire to quit. He states, "I will die soon anyway, why quit now?" On further review of his patient chart, it is noted that he has presented with the same chief complaint in the past and was diagnosed with acute bronchitis and treated with albuterol and antibiotics. He has not been to the office in over 3 years.

REVIEW OF SYSTEMS

The patient's ROS is positive for productive cough, wheezing, SOB, fatigue, dyspnea on exertion, crackles, and clubbing of fingernails. His ROS is negative for fever, chills, adenopathy, cyanosis, pallor, palpitations, or barrel chest.

RELEVANT HISTORY

The patient has medically uncontrolled hypertension and hyperlipidemia. He has been using albuterol and beclomethasone dipropionate inhaler occasionally for his SOB. He is not sure why he takes them. He denies having a history of asthma. He is a smoker. He has not received his flu vaccine for the last few years. He is not sure if he has ever had a pneumonia vaccine. He drinks about six 12 ounce beers three times a week. He is retired but used to work as an auto mechanic. No surgical history is reported. He does not know his family history.

ALLERGIES

No known drug allergies; no known food allergies.

MEDICATIONS

- Lisinopril 20 mg, QD
- Atorvastatin 20 mg, QD
- Albuterol 90 mcg inhaler, two puffs via inhalation q4h PRN for chest tightness or cough.
- Beclomethasone dipropionate 80 mg inhaler, two puffs via inhalation q12h.
- Ibuprofen 600 mg OTC, PRN for general aches.
- Guaifenesin cough syrup OTC, 15 mL q6h PRN for cough.

PHYSICAL EXAMINATION

Vitals: T 36.6°C (97.9°F), P 85, R 20, BP 152/88, SpO$_2$ 93%, HT 180.3 cm (71 in.), WT 84.8 kg (187 lbs), BMI 26.1.

General: Appears to be in mild respiratory distress due to accessory muscle usage for breathing, not tripoding. Noted a thin body habitus.

Psychiatric: Normal affect and judgment on exam.

Skin, Hair, and Nails: Mild clubbing of nails noted. No pallor or cyanosis present.

ENT/Mouth: Pink and moist oropharyngeal mucosa without exudates or lesions.

Neck: Supple, no adenopathy noted.

Lungs: Diffuse wheezing and crackles noted in both upper and lower lung fields. Labored breathing with accessory muscle usage noted; symmetrical expansion of lungs noted. Increased resonance to percussion noted. Decreased breath sounds throughout.

Heart: RRR; no murmur or gallops.

Neurologic: A&O×3, no focal deficit on exam noted.

CLINICAL DISCUSSION QUESTIONS

1. What is the differential diagnosis?

_____

_____

_____

_____

2. What is the most likely diagnosis? Why?

_____

_____

_____

_____

3. Demonstrate your understanding about the pathophysiology in regard to the most likely diagnosis.

_____

_____

_____

_____

4. Should tests/imaging studies be ordered? Which ones? Why? Think about tests/imaging beyond the primary care setting as well.

_____

_____

_____

_____

_____

5. What are the next appropriate steps in management?

_____

_____

_____

_____

6. Review recent and credible research articles on this diagnosis. What is a common misdiagnosis and what are initial treatment options? Provide references for your response.

_____

_____

_____

_____

_____

7. What are the pertinent ICD-10 and CPT (E/M) codes for this visit? Provide a short rationale.

_____

_____

_____

_____

8. What is the appropriate patient education for this case?

_____

_____

_____

_____

9. If not managed appropriately, what is/are the medical/legal concern(s) that may arise?

_____

_____

_____

_____

10. Think about interprofessional collaboration for this case. Provide a list of specialties or other disciplines and indicate what contribution these professionals might make to managing the patient.

_____

_____

_____

_____

BEDSIDE MANNER QUESTION

11. What would your communication style/approach be with this patient?

_____

_____

_____

_____

_____

ANSWER KEY *available at*
https://connect.springerpub.com/content/book/978-0-8261-8273-9

CHIEF COMPLAINT

"Fatigue and joint aches."

HISTORY OF PRESENT ILLNESS

A 55-year-old man presents to a free clinic complaining of fatigue, headache, and muscle and joint aches. The patient states he was seen at the clinic 1 month ago with the same symptoms and was diagnosed with a viral infection and instructed in supportive care, including oral hydration and acetaminophen. The symptoms began 2 to 3 months ago. He thinks he has a fever but has not checked the temperature. Aspirin has not helped. His muscle and joint aches are diffuse. There is no joint swelling or erythema. His headache is in the temple and occipital region, the pain is constant, and the patient denies photo or phonophobia. He denies any recent injuries and has no sick contacts.

REVIEW OF SYSTEMS

The ROS is positive for a 15-lb weight loss over the past 2 months and swollen lymph nodes in his groin and armpits. The ROS was negative for chills, sweats, nausea and vomiting, rash, SOB, chest pain, abdominal pain, or weakness.

RELEVANT HISTORY

The patient's medical history is positive for hypertension that is presently untreated. He has no surgical history. His social history includes consuming an occasional beer, but he denies smoking or IV drug abuse. The patient worked as an accountant but lost his job 5 years ago. He lives in a homeless shelter and works as a janitor. His family history is positive for mother dying at age 65 due to renal failure as a complication of diabetes; his father died at age 72 from a MI. His brothers are alive and well at ages 60 and 58.

ALLERGIES

No known drug allergies; no known food allergies.

MEDICATIONS

Acetaminophen 500 mg every 6 hours PRN for fever.

PHYSICAL EXAMINATION

Vitals: T 38.1°C (100.6°F), P 102, R 20, BP 149/89, WT 61.7 kg (136 lbs), HT 177.8 cm (70 in.), BMI 19.5.

General: A 55-year-old man who appears older than his stated age; he appears tired, thin, and without energy.

Psychiatric: Appears tired but no signs of depression or anxiety.

Skin, Hair, and Nails: Skin is warm and dry; fingernails are smooth and shiny, transparent, and normally curved. Hair distribution shows male pattern baldness; remaining hair is thick with normal luster.

Eyes: Corneas are clear. Conjunctivas are moist and without discharge; small red spots are seen on conjunctiva. Disc margins are sharp, arterioles are bright red with a narrow light reflex, and there is no tapering or nicking noted. There are no hemorrhages or exudates.

ENT/Mouth: Auricles are non-tender. Canals are patent; the tympanic membranes are intact; no bulging or erythema is noted.

Neck: There is no swelling or tenderness noted in the pre- or post-auricular nodes and posterior cervical, anterior cervical, or supraclavicular nodes.

Lungs: Breath sounds are heard throughout the lungs; are symmetric and vesicular. Breath sounds are low pitched and of soft intensity. No adventitious sounds are noted.

Heart: RRR. There is a grade IV/VI holosystolic murmur in the mitral region that radiates to the left axilla; a loud S3 and audible S4.

Abdomen: On inspection, the abdomen is symmetric; skin is smooth and soft without striae. No bulges, peristalsis, or pulsations are visible. On auscultation, clicks and gurgles are heard 10 to 15 times per minute; no hums, bruits, or friction rubs are heard. On percussions, the liver size is 6 cm midsternal line and 9 cm midclavicular line. There is no tenderness on light or deep palpation. The spleen tip can be palpated 2 cm below the costal margin on deep inspiration. There is no tenderness to light or deep palpation. No referred pain or rebound tenderness.

Lymphatic: There are several tender lymph nodes in the axilla bilaterally and there are moderate-sized, tender inguinal lymph nodes bilaterally.

Musculoskeletal: There are no areas of heat, tenderness, or soft tissue thickening; no fluid in the joints. Some tenderness is noted with movement of the knees.

Neurologic: A&O×3; cranial nerves II to XII are grossly intact.

CLINICAL DISCUSSION QUESTIONS

1. What is the differential diagnosis?

_____

_____

_____

_____

2. What is the most likely diagnosis? Why?

_____

_____

_____

_____

3. Demonstrate your understanding about the pathophysiology in regard to the most likely diagnosis.

_____

_____

_____

4. Should tests/imaging studies be ordered? Which ones? Why? Think about tests/imaging beyond the primary care setting as well.

_____

_____

_____

_____

5. What are the next appropriate steps in management?

_____

_____

_____

_____

6. What are the causes, risk factors, diagnosis, and treatments of the diagnosis? Provide references for your response.

_____

_____

_____

_____

7. What are the pertinent ICD-10 and CPT (E/M) codes for this visit? Provide a short rationale.

_____

_____

_____

_____

8. What is the appropriate patient education for this case?

_____

_____

_____

_____

9. If not managed appropriately, what is/are the medical/legal concern(s) that may arise?

_____

_____

_____

_____

10. Think about interprofessional collaboration for this case. Provide a list of specialties or other disciplines and indicate what contribution these professionals might make to managing the patient.

_____

_____

_____

_____

BEDSIDE MANNER QUESTION
11. What would your communication style/approach be with this patient?

_____

_____

_____

_____

ANSWER KEY _available at_
https://connect.springerpub.com/content/book/978-0-8261-8273-9

SHOULDER PAIN, ADULT MALE

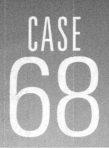

CHIEF COMPLAINT
"Shoulder pain."

HISTORY OF PRESENT ILLNESS
A 26-year-old man presents to his PCP for ED follow-up. A firefighter, yesterday, nearly collapsed fighting a fire. He was in full gear and fighting fires from early in the morning "non-stop." He states he tried to stay hydrated and drank a lot of water during the day but started feeling "lightheaded and woozy" and he asked to take a break. They were cutting a fire line requiring rigorous digging, shoveling, and cutting brush. After taking a short 15-minute break he resumed to his usual duties only to sit back out roughly 20 minutes later due to severe muscle pain in his calves and shoulders. He tried to continue but the pain was too severe. He informed his captain who transported him to the closest ED for evaluation. The local ED evaluated him and informed him he was dehydrated. He was told that his urine was very dark and was encouraged to drink fluids and was released. The patient states, "I continue to see dark colored urine." He called in sick this morning because of the pain mostly in his shoulders and an overall feeling "like I've been hit by a truck."

REVIEW OF SYSTEMS
The patient's ROS is positive for weakness and exhaustion, palpitations, SOB, nausea, dark-colored urine, and muscle pain in his shoulders, lower back, and calves. His ROS is negative for diarrhea, constipation, anuria, hematuria, muscle weakness, numbness, or tingling.

RELEVANT HISTORY
The patient's history is significant for multiple musculoskeletal injuries secondary to his occupation. These include shoulder injury and knee injury. His social history includes a beer on the weekend with no history of tobacco or other substance use. He is single. He has no children. His mother has a history of breast cancer (remission) and his father has no known medical illnesses. He has no siblings.

ALLERGIES
No known drug allergies; no known food allergies.

MEDICATIONS
None.

PHYSICAL EXAMINATION
Vitals: T 37.3°C (99.1°F), P 96, R 12, BP 134/86, HT 185.42 cm (73 in.), WT 102.05 kg (225 lbs), BMI 29.7.

General: A&O; no acute distress. Overweight.

Skin, Hair, and Nails: No erythema or pallor of skin noted. Hair and nails showed no abnormal findings.

Head: Normocephalic.

Eyes: PERRL.

ENT/Mouth: Mucous membranes moist and pink.

Neck: Supple; no masses; normal thyroid; no jugular vein distension.

Lungs: Vesicular breath sounds diffusely. Breath sounds were equal throughout.

Heart: RRR; no murmurs, rubs, or gallops; nondisplaced PMI. Capillary refill less than 2 seconds.

Abdomen: Soft; mild epigastric tenderness; no costovertebral angle tenderness; no splenomegaly; no hepatomegaly. Tenderness with palpation generalized over bilateral flanks.

Musculoskeletal: Generalized tenderness to palpation over bilateral shoulders. Limited ROM of shoulders bilaterally due to pain. Generalized tenderness over calves and quadriceps bilaterally. There is severe pain over palpation a paralumbar musculature with voluntary guarding and hypertonicity.

Neurology: A&O×3. Cranial nerves II to XII intact.

CLINICAL DISCUSSION QUESTIONS

1. What is the differential diagnosis?

_____

_____

_____

_____

2. What is the most likely diagnosis? Why?

_____

_____

_____

_____

3. Demonstrate your understanding about the pathophysiology in regard to the most likely diagnosis.

_____

_____

_____

_____

4. Should tests/imaging studies be ordered? Which ones? Why? Think about tests/imaging beyond the primary care setting as well.

_____

_____

_____

_____

5. What are the next appropriate steps in management?

_____

_____

_____

_____

6. What are the complications and most common cause of the diagnosis? Provide references for your response.

_____

_____

_____

_____

7. What are the pertinent ICD-10 and CPT (E/M) codes for this visit? Provide a short rationale.

_____

_____

_____

_____

8. What is the appropriate patient education for this case?

_____

_____

_____

_____

9. If not managed appropriately, what is/are the medical/legal concern(s) that may arise?

_____

_____

_____

_____

10. Think about interprofessional collaboration for this case. Provide a list of specialties or other disciplines and indicate what contribution these professionals might make to managing the patient.

_____

_____

_____

_____

BEDSIDE MANNER QUESTIONS

11. What would your communication style/approach be with this patient?

_____

_____

_____

_____

12. If a patient is distressed by the diagnosis, what might offer support?

_____

_____

_____

_____

ANSWER KEY *available at*
https://connect.springerpub.com/content/book/978-0-8261-8273-9

CHIEF COMPLAINT

"Unexplained weight loss."

HISTORY OF PRESENT ILLNESS

A 36-year-old woman presents to her PCP with multiple complaints: weight loss and palpitations worsened by anxiety about her health for the last 3 months. She states she has been the sole care-taker for her ill mother for the last 6 months and had no time for herself or time to seek care. She states she was noticing a weight loss of 15 pounds continuing even though she has been indulging nervous eating habits especially when she is stressed. The patient states she is stressed and anxious about her health after witnessing how Alzheimer's is affecting her mother. The patient attributes her palpitations to anxiety about her health and her mother's health.

REVIEW OF SYSTEMS

A ROS was positive for weight loss, palpitations, and anxiety. The ROS was negative for sweating, heat intolerance, tremors, headache, change of vision, chest pain, SOB, fever, chills, vomiting, diarrhea, constipation, or suicidal ideation.

RELEVANT HISTORY

The patient's history is significant for a negative screening of depression and anxiety done last year during a physical exam. She is not a smoker. She has a 12-pack year smoking history, but quit 5 years ago. There is no substance abuse history (including both alcohol and drugs). She is sexually active and in a monogamous relationship with her husband of 10 years. She reports she is happy with her husband and children. Her family history is positive for diabetes, hypertension, and CAD.

ALLERGIES

No known drug allergies; no known food allergies.

MEDICATIONS

Melatonin 4 mg PRN for sleep.

PHYSICAL EXAMINATION

Vitals: T 37.2°C (98.9°F), P 102, R 18, BP 130/78, WT 101.6 kg (224 lbs), HT 170 cm (67 in.), BMI 35.
General: Appears anxious and fatigued; mild acute distress.
Psychiatric: Mildly anxious, scored negative on PHQ9 and GAD7.

Eyes: Mild exophthalmos with reactive and responsive pupils with light, intact extraocular movements. Bilateral conjunctival inflammation noted.

Neck: Soft, non-tender, slightly and diffusely enlarged thyroid without lymphadenopathy.

Heart: Tachycardic, S1 and S2 present without murmur or gallop.

Lungs: Clear to auscultation bilaterally, good air movement throughout.

Abdomen: Soft, non-distended, and moderately tender throughout.

Extremities: No bilateral swelling.

Neurologic: A&O×3, cranial nerves II to XII intact.

CLINICAL DISCUSSION QUESTIONS

1. What is the differential diagnosis?

_____

_____

_____

_____

2. What is the most likely diagnosis? Why?

_____

_____

_____

_____

3. Demonstrate your understanding about the pathophysiology in regard to the most likely diagnosis.

_____

_____

_____

_____

4. Should tests/imaging studies be ordered? Which ones? Why? Think about tests/imaging beyond the primary care setting as well.

_____

_____

_____

_____

5. What are the next appropriate steps in management?

_____

_____

_____

_____

6. What are the cause and clinical manifestations of the diagnosis? Provide references for your response.

_____

_____

_____

_____

7. What are the pertinent ICD-10 and CPT (E/M) codes for this visit? Provide a short rationale.

_____

_____

_____

_____

8. What is the appropriate patient education for this case?

_____

_____

_____

_____

9. If not managed appropriately, what is/are the medical/legal concern(s) that may arise?

_____

_____

_____

_____

10. Think about interprofessional collaboration for this case. Provide a list of specialties or other disciplines and indicate what contribution these professionals might make to managing the patient.

_____

_____

_____

_____

BEDSIDE MANNER QUESTIONS

11. What would your communication style/approach be with this patient?

_____

_____

_____

12. If a patient is distressed by the diagnosis, what might offer support?

_____

_____

_____

_____

ANSWER KEY _available at_
https://connect.springerpub.com/content/book/978-0-8261-8273-9

LIGHTHEADEDNESS, GERIATRIC FEMALE

CHIEF COMPLAINT
"Lightheadedness."

HISTORY OF PRESENT ILLNESS
A 68-year-old-woman with a medical history of essential hypertension presents to her PCP with generalized weakness and lightheadedness. She states she has been overall unwell for the past 3 days. She is weak to the point she has a hard time doing the usual tasks around the house. The patient states she has been lying down for most of the past 2 days. When she gets up and walks around, she is intermittently lightheaded. She is overall active and usually enjoys working in her garden, but the past few days she has been unable to do much due to the fatigue and lightheadedness. The patient is generally adherent with her medications, which include hydrochlorothiazide 25 mg PO daily and amlodipine 5 mg PO daily. She is accompanied by her daughter who has reported that in addition to the fatigue, her mother has had a lack of appetite and decreased oral intake over the past 2 days.

REVIEW OF SYSTEMS
A directed ROS is positive for fatigue, fevers, chills, left-sided flank pain, dysuria, and urinary frequency. Her ROS is negative for headaches, visual disturbances, nasal congestion, sore throat, palpitations, chest pain, abdomen pain, nausea/vomiting, focal weakness or numbness, confusion, weight gain or loss, polyphagia or polydipsia, anxiety, or depression.

RELEVANT HISTORY
The patient's history is significant for essential hypertension diagnosed at age 52; her social history is negative for drug, tobacco, or alcohol use. She reports a family history of hypertension and high cholesterol. The patient lives at home with her husband, they have been married for 33 years, and she describes her marriage and family life as happy and healthy. She has two children both grown-up and living on their own.

ALLERGIES
No known allergies; no known food allergies.

MEDICATIONS
- Hydrochlorothiazide 25 mg PO QD
- Amlodipine 5 mg PO QD

PHYSICAL EXAMINATION
Vitals: T 38.8°C (102°F), P 106, R 18, BP 88/30, HT 165.10 cm (65 in.), WT 61.2 kg (135 lbs), BMI 22.5.

General: Patient is in no apparent distress, appears stated age.

Psychiatric: Normal affect, no disorganized behavior.

Skin, Hair, and Nails: No rashes, normal skin turgor, normal hair texture, nails without splinter hemorrhages or clubbing.

Head: Normocephalic, atraumatic, no lesions.

Eyes: PERRL, anicteric sclerae.

ENT/Mouth: Mucous membranes dry, no oral cavity lesions, oropharynx without erythema.

Neck: Normal neck circumference, no thyromegaly.

Chest: No obvious pectus deformity, normal excursion.

Lungs: Unlabored respirations, clear to auscultation bilaterally.

Heart: RRR, no murmurs, S1 and S2 present with normal timing.

Abdomen: No striae, soft, non-tender, bowel sounds are present and normoactive.

Musculoskeletal: Left-sided CVA tenderness.

Neurologic: A&O×3, cranial nerves II to XII intact, motor strength is 5/5 at the upper extremity and lower extremity bilaterally, no gross sensory deficits.

CLINICAL DISCUSSION QUESTIONS

1. What is the differential diagnosis?

_____

_____

_____

2. What is the most likely diagnosis? Why?

_____

_____

_____

_____

3. Demonstrate your understanding about the pathophysiology in regard to the most likely diagnosis.

_____

_____

_____

_____

4. Should tests/imaging studies be ordered? Which ones? Why? Think about tests/imaging beyond the primary care setting as well.

_____

_____

_____

_____

5. What are the next appropriate steps in management?

_____

_____

_____

_____

6. Review a reliable, recent reference and demonstrate diagnostic criteria and treatment approach associated with this diagnosis. Include the name of the reference.

_____

_____

_____

_____

7. What are the pertinent ICD-10 and CPT (E/M) codes for this visit? Provide a short rationale.

_____

_____

_____

_____

8. What is the appropriate patient education for this case?

_____

_____

_____

_____

9. If not managed appropriately, what is/are the medical/legal concern(s) that may arise?

_____

_____

_____

_____

10. Think about interprofessional collaboration for this case. Provide a list of specialties or other disciplines and indicate what contribution these professionals might make to managing the patient.

_____

_____

_____

_____

BEDSIDE MANNER QUESTION

11. What would your communication/style approach be with this patient?

_____

_____

_____

_____

ANSWER KEY *available at*
https://connect.springerpub.com/content/book/978-0-8261-8273-9

PAINFUL LUMP IN ARMPIT, ADULT FEMALE

CHIEF COMPLAINT

"Painful lump in armpit."

HISTORY OF PRESENT ILLNESS

A 23-year-old woman with no significant medical history is brought to her PCP by her boyfriend who is worried about "a really painful lump in her armpit that is not going away." The patient states she noticed a small, rubbery bump that appeared in the center of her left axilla approximately 4 days ago. She thought a pimple was developing as she reports noticing them periodically after shaving with her boyfriend's razor. This one, she states, is getting larger, seems to be spreading, and is very painful.

She reports slight chills and a fever that started this morning but has not taken her temperature. She admits to a stinging, burning 9/10 pain in her left axilla, extending into her left inner elbow with any movement of her left upper extremity. She denies numbness or tingling of her left hand and fingers. Being right-hand dominant, she reports trying not to use her left arm as the pain intensifies with movement, especially noticed when trying to apply deodorant today. She has tried over-the-counter ibuprofen which she states has helped little to reduce the pain that is interfering with her sleep. Her last dose of two 200 mg tablets was at 11 p.m. last night. She does not recall when her last tetanus immunization was, neither can she recall that this issue has ever been this worrisome before. She denies exposure to new perfumes, colognes, soaps, detergents, or dyes.

REVIEW OF SYSTEMS

The patient's ROS is positive for subjective fever, chills, fatigue, and insomnia for 1 day due to painful left axilla. ROS is also positive for painful, erythematous mass in her left axilla for 4 days; pain extends to elbow, sparing left hand and fingers. Her ROS is negative for unintentional weight loss, weakness, numbness, tingling, or paralysis of left upper extremity.

RELEVANT HISTORY

The patient had acute appendicitis with a resultant laparoscopic appendectomy at age 17. Her last menstrual period was 2 months ago, menses four times per year secondary to birth control taken. She is a social smoker (5 to 6 cigarettes on weekends) and has 1 to 2 vodka/energy drinks per weekend. She denies recreational or illicit drug use. Her family history is noncontributory.

ALLERGIES

No known drug allergies; no known food allergies.

MEDICATIONS

- Extended-cycle birth control pills, one tablet daily
- Ibuprofen, two 200 mg tablets PO PRN left axillary pain

PHYSICAL EXAMINATION

Vitals: T 37.7°C (99.8°F), P 88, R 14, BP 128/72, HT 170.2 cm (67 in.), WT 62 kg (136 lbs), BMI 21.3.

General: A well-nourished young adult female of stated age is found sitting on the examination table in slight discomfort. She is A&O×3.

Skin, Hair, and Nails: Deeply seated, cord-like nodular and elongated 4 cm × 1 cm left axillary mass that is erythematous, tender, and swollen, extending distally to left anterior breast. Mass is slightly fluctuant at its center with multiple pointing white heads, diffusely warm. The skin surrounding the mass is slightly hard to palpation. No lacerations, open lesions, or drainage. No skin lesions or lacerations on any other area of the patient's body.

Neck: FROM, cervical and tonsillar lymphadenopathy, L > R.

Breasts: Firm, slightly pendulous, symmetric bilaterally, without nipple discharge or retraction. Tender left tail of Spence, extending proximally to erythematous left axillary mass.

Lungs: Clear to auscultation bilaterally, without wheezes.

Heart: RRR without murmurs, rubs, or gallops.

Peripheral Vascular: Extremities warm throughout, BUE and BLE pulses 2+ and symmetric. capillary refill brisk, less than 2 seconds throughout. Upper and lower distal extremities without edema. No varicosities.

Musculoskeletal: FROM of right upper extremity. LROM left shoulder, eliciting severe pain with left upper extremity extension overhead with external rotation. FROM left elbow, wrist, hand, and fingers.

Neurologic: Cranial nerves II to XII grossly intact. Upper and lower extremity sensation intact to light and sharp touch. Muscle bulk, tone, 5/5 strength symmetric throughout. Bilateral brachioradialis and patellar reflexes 2+/symmetric.

CLINICAL DISCUSSION QUESTIONS

1. What is the differential diagnosis?

_____

_____

_____

_____

2. What is the most likely diagnosis? Why?

_____

_____

_____

_____

3. Demonstrate your understanding about the pathophysiology in regard to the most likely diagnosis.

_____

_____

_____

_____

4. Should tests/imaging studies be ordered? Which ones? Why? Think about tests/imaging beyond the primary care setting as well.

_____

_____

_____

_____

5. What are the next appropriate steps in management?

_____

_____

_____

_____

6. What are the exacerbation factors, diagnosis, and treatment of the diagnosis? Provide references for your responses.

_____

_____

_____

_____

7. What are the pertinent ICD-10 and CPT (E/M) codes for this visit? Provide a short rationale.

_____

_____

_____

_____

8. What is the appropriate patient education for this case?

_____

_____

_____

_____

9. If not managed appropriately, what is/are the medical/legal concern(s) that may arise?

_____

_____

_____

_____

10. Think about interprofessional collaboration for this case. Provide a list of specialties or other disciplines and indicate what contribution these professionals might make to managing the patient.

_____

_____

_____

_____

BEDSIDE MANNER QUESTION
11. What would your communication style/approach be with this patient?

_____

_____

_____

_____

ANSWER KEY _available at_
https://connect.springerpub.com/content/book/978-0-8261-8273-9

FEVER, COUGH, AND RUNNY NOSE, PEDIATRIC FEMALE

CHIEF COMPLAINT

"Fever, cough, and runny nose."

HISTORY OF PRESENT ILLNESS

During summer season, a mother brings her 9-month-old daughter to her PCP for evaluation of fever, cough, and runny nose for the past week. The mother states her child's fever started off at 37.8°C (100°F), but for the past 2 days it has been fluctuating between 38°C to 39°C (102°F to 103°F). She has been alternating between acetaminophen and ibuprofen q4-6h. This brings the fever to 38.3°C (101°F). A dry intermittent cough has been present for the past 4 days and is negative for post-tussive emesis. Her runny nose has progressively been getting worse over the past 7 days and the discharge is green. She has a poor appetite but is drinking okay. The mother has not noticed the child pulling her ears or showing any discomfort with urination. There is no history of vomiting or diarrhea.

REVIEW OF SYSTEMS

The child's ROS is positive for fever, cough, runny nose, and a decrease in appetite. The ROS is negative for vomiting and diarrhea.

RELEVANT HISTORY

The child was born by a normal spontaneous vaginal delivery, without any complications. She is up to date with immunizations including influenza vaccines. The child lives with her parents, has two siblings, and attends daycare. Her father is a smoker, but smokes away from the house and the car. Family history includes father is prediabetic and mother is obese.

ALLERGIES

No known drug allergies; no known food allergies.

MEDICATIONS

- Acetaminophen 160/5 mL 1 tsp q4h PRN.
- Ibuprofen 100/5 mL 1 tsp q6h PRN.

PHYSICAL EXAMINATION

Vitals: T 39.3°C (102.7°F), P 130, R 28, BP 98/62, WT 10 kg (22 lbs) 75th percentile, HT 68.6 cm (27 in.) 50th percentile, BMI 21.2.

General: Slightly uncomfortable, but aware of her surroundings. Not toxic.

Skin, Hair, and Nails: Warm and pink. No abnormal findings with hair or nails.

ENT/Mouth: Right TM: bulging, dull red, landmarks not visible. Left TM: slightly pink with a positive light reflex. Nose: purulent drainage. OP: patent and moist.

Lungs: Coarse breath sounds, mostly transmitted from upper airway congestion. Negative for wheezing or rhonchi.

Heart: RRR. No murmur was appreciated.

Abdomen: Soft, non-tender, non-distended.

Neurologic: Alert and interactive.

CLINICAL DISCUSSION QUESTIONS

1. What is the differential diagnosis?

_____

_____

_____

_____

2. What is the most likely diagnosis? Why?

_____

_____

_____

_____

3. Demonstrate your understanding about the pathophysiology in regard to the most likely diagnosis.

_____

_____

_____

_____

4. Should tests/imaging studies be ordered? Which ones? Why? Think about tests/imaging beyond the primary care setting as well.

_____

_____

_____

_____

5. What are the next appropriate steps in management?

_____

_____

_____

_____

6. What are the prevalence, prevention, risk factors, and treatments of the diagnosis? Provide the references for your responses.

_____

_____

_____

_____

7. What are the pertinent ICD-10 and CPT (E/M) codes for this visit? Provide a short rationale.

_____

_____

_____

_____

8. What is the appropriate parent/patient education topics for this case?

_____

_____

_____

_____

9. If not managed appropriately, what is/are the medical/legal concern(s) that may arise?

_____

_____

_____

_____

10. Think about interprofessional collaboration for this case. Provide a list of specialties or other disciplines and indicate what contribution these professionals might make to managing the patient.

_____

_____

_____

_____

BEDSIDE MANNER QUESTION

11. What would your communication style/approach be with this parent/patient?

_____

_____

_____

_____

ANSWER KEY *available at*
https://connect.springerpub.com/content/book/978-0-8261-8273-9

DIABETES CHECK, ADULT MALE

CASE
73

CHIEF COMPLAINT
"Diabetes check."

HISTORY OF PRESENT ILLNESS

A 58-year-old Hispanic man presents to a new PCP to check on his diabetes status. His last annual visit was almost 3 years ago, and it has been 6 months since his last diabetes visit. The patient also states he used to see a "specialist for his kidney" but stopped going and wants to initiate care here due to his insurance. He was diagnosed with diabetes almost 5 years ago (cannot recall exact years), and he has been taking metformin 500 mg BID for his diabetes most of the days (he forgets some days). For his high cholesterol, he has been taking atorvastatin 40 mg daily. He was also told he has high BP. He was started on a medication for his BP but stopped taking because he felt OK. The patient admits he does not keep appointments well and he used to be on insulin prior; however, he was not adherent. He states cost as the barrier that kept him from adhering to his medication regimen. He now has active insurance. His diet consists of red meats, fast food, rice, beans, and potatoes. He also complains of chronic fatigue and headaches that are intermittent but occur more frequently now and are worse in severity. The headache located in the occipital region and radiates to the temporal regions. The patient describes the pain as a throbbing and pulsating sensation. He notes some eye blurriness and nausea at times and thinks he drinks more than what he voids but has no difficulty voiding.

REVIEW OF SYSTEMS

The patient's ROS is positive for fatigue, nausea, urine retention, and occipital headache. Pertinent negatives are aura, vomiting, sudden vision changes, or loss or halos. He denies cognitive problems, angina, SOB, diaphoresis, palpitations, or extremity swelling. He further denies polydipsia, polyphagia, polyuria dysuria, hematuria, discharge, hesitancy, frequency, or dribbling.

RELEVANT HISTORY

The patient's history is significant for hypertension, type 2 DM, and hyperlipidemia. He has a family history of HTN, DM (type unknown), and hyperlipidemia. He is a field worker, is married, and has two children.

ALLERGIES

No known drug allergies; no known food allergies.

MEDICATION

Metformin 500 mg BID
Atorvastatin 40 mg QD

PHYSICAL EXAMINATION

Vitals: T 36.8°C (98.2°F), P 92, R 16, BP 178/106, HT 170.18 cm (67 in.), WT 83 kg (183 lbs), BMI 28.66.

General: Alert, well hydrated, in no distress, well developed, well nourished.

Psychiatric: Cognitive function intact, cooperative with exam, good eye contact.

Eyes: EOMI, PERRLA.

Neck: Supple, FROM, no cervical lymphadenopathy, no thyromegaly.

Chest: Normal shape and expansion.

Lungs: Clear to auscultation bilaterally, good air movement.

Heart: RRR, no jugular vein distention or murmurs.

Abdomen: Active bowel sounds ×4, no distention, nontender with no rebound, soft on palpation.

Musculoskeletal: Mild pitting edema bilaterally 1+, pedal pulses 2+ bilaterally, no clubbing, cyanosis.

Neurologic: Nonfocal, A&O×3, normal gait. Cranial nerves II to XII grossly intact.

CLINICAL DISCUSSION QUESTIONS

1. What is the differential diagnosis?

_____

_____

_____

_____

2. What is the most likely diagnosis? Why?

_____

_____

_____

_____

3. Demonstrate your understanding about the pathophysiology in regard to the most likely diagnosis.

_____

_____

_____

_____

4. Should tests/imaging studies be ordered? Which ones? Why? Think about tests/imaging beyond the primary care setting as well.

_____

_____

_____

_____

5. What are the next appropriate steps in management?

_____

_____

_____

_____

6. Using credible literature, explain whether Hispanic patients are at a greater or lesser risk for this diagnosis and why. Provide references for your responses.

_____

_____

_____

_____

7. What are the pertinent ICD-10 and CPT (E/M) codes for this visit? Provide a short rationale.

_____

_____

_____

_____

8. What is the appropriate patient education for this case?

_____

_____

_____

_____

9. If not managed appropriately, what is/are the medical/legal concern(s) that may arise?

_____

_____

_____

_____

10. Think about interprofessional collaboration for this case. Provide a list of specialties or other disciplines and indicate what contribution these professionals might make to managing the patient.

_____

_____

_____

_____

BEDSIDE MANNER QUESTIONS

11. What would your communication style/approach be with this patient?

_____

_____

_____

_____

12. If a patient is distressed by the diagnosis, what might offer support?

_____

_____

_____

_____

ANSWER KEY _available at_
https://connect.springerpub.com/content/book/978-0-8261-8273-9

BUTTOCKS PAIN, GERIATRIC MALE

CHIEF COMPLAINT

"Buttocks pain."

HISTORY OF PRESENT ILLNESS

A 67-year-old man presents to establish care as a new patient. He has hypertension, type 2 DM, hyperlipidemia, and mental retardation for which he has been off medication for 6 months. He complains of buttocks pain for a few days. He denies any falls.

He is living with his disabled sister and niece who have taken care of him for the last few years after they removed him from a residential facility due to cost. He was in a program that provided sheltered work experience and socialization. His niece is the patient's payee and manages his financial and medical needs; however, she has not taken him to a doctor for over 6 months and is not keeping him adherent to his medical regimen.

The patient's last HbA1C was 8.6% over 6 months ago, and he does not have a glucometer for BG monitoring. The dates of his last eye exam or dental exam are unknown.

His sister has limited ability to help the patient meet his medical and physical needs due to her medical condition. The niece is not interested in home health services. She uses the patient's and her mother's disability checks to pay for bills and does not have money left for medications.

The patient states he washes dishes and watches TV during the day for his activities. He is able to bathe and toilet himself with prompting and assistance. He uses a walker for stability with ambulation. He is missing his glasses and dentures due to frequent moves over the last few years.

REVIEW OF SYSTEMS

The patient's ROS is positive for weight loss of 20 lbs, missing teeth, poor visual acuity, right shoulder pain with movement, right foot drop, and weakness. His ROS is negative for fever, chills, fatigue, vomiting, diarrhea, polyuria, polydipsia, and polyphagia. All other ROS are negative.

RELEVANT HISTORY

The patient's history is significant for intellectual disability, type 2 diabetes, hypertension, hyperlipidemia, right foot drop, and nearsightedness. He had a full dental extraction in 2013. He lives with his sister, niece, and his niece's three children. He does not drink alcohol or use tobacco products or illicit drugs.

ALLERGIES

No known drug allergies; no known food allergies.

MEDICATIONS

- Enalapril 20 mg PO BID.
- Glipizide 5 mg PO BID.
- Metformin 1000 mg PO BID.
- Metoprolol tartrate 50 mg PO BID.
- Pravastatin 40 mg PO QD.

PHYSICAL EXAMINATION

Vitals: T 37°C (98.6°F), P 88, R 16, BP 180/100, HT 185.4 cm (6'1"), WT 126.6 kg (279 lbs), BMI 36.81.

General: Well-developed, malnourished appearing 67-year-old man in acute distress. Poor hygiene with dirty clothes and foul body odor. Able to answer questions.

Psychiatric: Normal mood.

Skin, Hair, and Nails: Dry appearing, macerated, erythematous skin on buttocks and gluteal fold with dry fecal material. Partial thickness, loss of dermis with shallow ulceration on left buttocks. Dirty, long fingernails. Toenails are thickened and yellow with extensive growth needing trimming to normal length.

ENT/Mouth: Dry oral mucosa, teeth are absent, no dentures.

Lungs: Clear to auscultation bilaterally.

Heart: RRR, without murmur, gallop, or rub.

Abdomen: Soft, non-distended. Normoactive bowel sounds are heard in all four quadrants.

Musculoskeletal: No joint swelling or pain. Wide gait with dragging of right foot.

Neurologic: Coordination abnormal with drop foot pattern of right foot. Sensory exam of the foot is abnormal with monofilaments in all locations. Weak pulses, no lesions, or ulcers. Mini-cog was normal.

CLINICAL DISCUSSION QUESTIONS

1. What is the differential diagnosis?

_____

_____

_____

_____

2. What is the most likely diagnosis? Why?

_____

_____

_____

_____

3. Demonstrate your understanding about the pathophysiology in regard to the most likely diagnosis.

_____

_____

_____

_____

4. Should tests/imaging studies be ordered? Which ones? Why? Think about tests/imaging beyond the primary care setting as well.

_____

_____

_____

_____

5. What are the next appropriate steps in management?

_____

_____

_____

_____

6. What are the risk factors, clinical presentation, and PCP responsibility associated with the diagnosis? Provide references for your response.

_____

_____

_____

_____

7. What are the pertinent ICD-10 and CPT (E/M) codes for this visit? Provide a short rationale.

_____

_____

_____

_____

8. What are appropriate patient/caregiver education topics for this case?

_____

_____

_____

_____

9. If not managed appropriately, what is/are the medical/legal concern(s) that may arise?

_____

_____

_____

_____

10. Think about interprofessional collaboration for this case. Provide a list of specialties or other disciplines and indicate what contribution these professionals might make to managing the patient and family.

_____

_____

_____

_____

BEDSIDE MANNER QUESTION
11. What would your communication style/approach be with this family?

_____

_____

_____

_____

ANSWER KEY _available at_
https://connect.springerpub.com/content/book/978-0-8261-8273-9

ABDOMINAL PAIN, ADOLESCENT MALE

CHIEF COMPLAINT
"Abdominal pain."

HISTORY OF PRESENT ILLNESS
A 14-year-old boy presents to his PCP with abdominal pain that has been ongoing for 1 week. His foster mother is unable to pinpoint any particular symptom that stands out. He has no complaints of nausea, vomiting, diarrhea, or fever. He denies any aggravating or relieving factors. He does not eat spicy food, eats chocolate only occasionally, and doesn't skip meals. He drinks soda and orange juice occasionally. He does not drink coffee. He is unable to localize the pain. The consistency of his stool is soft. His appetite has decreased. He adds that he unable to sleep at night and is not sure why. His body language and the tone of his voice at this juncture see, as though he is scared and anxious about something. To put him at ease, the remainder of the history is taken with a chaperone and the foster mother is requested to step from the room. When asked if there is anything else that he would like to share, he opens up about what happened 2 months ago at a party. "It was a wild party, and everyone was hooking up." He really didn't know anyone there but ended up "hooking up" with a girl he just met. He wanted to fit in at the party and is now worried that he may have caught something. He denies any penile discharge or dysuria.

REVIEW OF SYSTEMS
The patient's ROS is positive for anxiety, anorexia, insomnia, and abdominal pain. His ROS was negative for nausea, vomiting, diarrhea, constipation, fever, rash, and dysuria.

RELEVANT HISTORY
The patient has no chronic conditions and hospitalizations. His immunizations are up to date. He is in middle school and lives with a foster mother and three other foster children at home. His family history is unknown.

ALLERGIES
No known drug allergies; no known food allergies.

MEDICATIONS
None.

PHYSICAL EXAMINATION
Vitals: T 37.0°C (98.7°F), P 100, R 20, BP 110/68, WT 50.8 kg (112 lbs), HT 162.6 cm (64 in.), BMI 19.2.

General: Alert and not in any distress.

Psychiatric: Anxious.

Skin, Hair, and Nails: Jaundice +. No signs of nail-biting or cuts on the wrist. No rash. No abnormal findings with hair or nails.

Eyes: Red reflex intact. PERRL. No icterus.

Abdomen: Non-tender and soft on palpation. Not distended. Bowel sounds are normal. No organomegaly or masses.

Genital/Rectal: Normal penile and scrotal exam. No skin lesions noted. Rectal exam was deferred.

Neurologic: A&O×3.

CLINICAL DISCUSSION QUESTIONS

1. What is the differential diagnosis?

_____

_____

_____

_____

2. What is the most likely diagnosis? Why?

_____

_____

_____

3. Demonstrate your understanding about the pathophysiology in regard to the most likely diagnosis.

_____

_____

_____

_____

4. Should tests/imaging studies be ordered? Which ones? Why? Think about tests/imaging beyond the primary care setting as well.

_____

_____

_____

_____

5. What are the next appropriate steps in management?

_____

_____

_____

_____

6. What are the prevalence, transmission, and screening of the diagnosis? Provide references for your response.

_____

_____

_____

_____

7. What are the pertinent ICD-10 and CPT (E/M) codes for this visit? Provide a short rationale.

_____

_____

_____

_____

8. What is the appropriate patient education for this case?

_____

_____

_____

_____

9. If not managed appropriately, what is/are the medical/legal concern(s) that may arise?

_____

_____

_____

_____

10. Think about interprofessional collaboration for this case. Provide a list of specialties or other disciplines and indicate what contribution these professionals might make to managing the patient.

_____

_____

_____

_____

BEDSIDE MANNER QUESTIONS

11. What would your communication style/approach be with this patient?

_____

_____

_____

_____

12. If a patient or his guardian is distressed by the diagnosis, what might offer support?

_____

_____

_____

_____

ANSWER KEY _available at_
https://connect.springerpub.com/content/book/978-0-8261-8273-9

IRRITABLE AND CRYING TODDLER, PEDIATRIC MALE

CHIEF COMPLAINT

"Irritable and crying toddler."

HISTORY OF PRESENT ILLNESS

A mother presents with her 16-month-old son to his PCP for an evaluation of irritability and crying for the past 5 hours. According to his mother, the child was fine, when suddenly became fussy and appeared to be in pain. He has no nausea, vomiting, diarrhea, fever, cough, or cold symptoms. His mother was alarmed by the sudden off-on episodes of crying. She explains that when he has short bursts of excruciating pain he doubles over or if he is being held his legs have pull up to his chest. The child seems to be fine in between these episodes. Typically, the child is calm.

REVIEW OF SYSTEMS

The patient's ROS is positive for irritability and possible abdominal pain. His ROS is negative for nausea, vomiting, bloody stool, constipation, fever, chills, and cough.

RELEVANT HISTORY

The child was a normal spontaneous vaginal delivery at term without any complications. He has continued to thrive hitting all developmental milestones. He has not been hospitalized neither is he on any chronic medications.

ALLERGIES

No known drug allergies; no known food allergies.

MEDICATIONS

None.

PHYSICAL EXAMINATION

Vitals: T 37.0°C (98.6°F), P 120, R 28, BP 100/65, WT 9.9 kg (22 lbs) 10th percentile, HT 76.2 cm (30 in.) 5th percentile, BMI 16.5.

General: Alert and engaging when not having an episode of pain. He is non-toxic looking.

Psychiatric: Irritable.

Skin, Hair, and Nails: Pink with a 1–2-second capillary refill. No abnormal findings with hair or nails.

Head: No signs of trauma.

Eyes: PERRL.

ENT/Mouth: Moist oral mucosa with no signs of dehydration.

Neck: FROM with no nuchal rigidity.

Lungs: Clear to auscultation bilaterally, equal breath sounds.

Heart: RRR, no murmurs.

Abdomen: Soft and non-distended. Mild tenderness with fullness in the right upper abdomen. The right lower abdomen is scaphoid and feels "empty" on palpation (Dance sign).

Genital/Rectal: Genital exam without abnormal finding; stool is hemoccult negative.

Neurologic: Alert and not lethargic.

CLINICAL DISCUSSION QUESTIONS

1. What is the differential diagnosis?

_____

_____

_____

_____

2. What is the most likely diagnosis? Why?

_____

_____

_____

_____

3. Demonstrate your understanding about the pathophysiology in regard to the most likely diagnosis.

_____

_____

_____

_____

4. Should tests/imaging studies be ordered? Which ones? Why? Think about tests/imaging beyond the primary care setting as well.

_____

_____

_____

_____

5. What are the next appropriate steps in management?

_____

_____

_____

_____

6. What is a cost-effective and highly specific diagnostic method for this diagnosis? What are the treatment options of this diagnosis? Provide references for your responses.

_____

_____

_____

_____

7. What are the pertinent ICD-10 and CPT (E/M) codes for this visit? Provide a short rationale.

_____

_____

_____

_____

8. What is the appropriate parent education for this case?

_____

_____

_____

_____

9. If not managed appropriately, what is/are the medical/legal concern(s) that may arise?

_____

_____

_____

_____

10. Think about interprofessional collaboration for this case. Provide a list of specialties or other disciplines and indicate what contribution these professionals might make to managing the patient.

_____

_____

_____

_____

BEDSIDE MANNER QUESTIONS

11. What would your communication style/approach be with this parent/patient?

_____

_____

_____

12. If a patient's parent is distressed by the diagnosis, what might offer support?

_____

_____

_____

_____

ANSWER KEY _available at_
https://connect.springerpub.com/content/book/978-0-8261-8273-9

SWELLING AROUND EYES AND ANKLES, ADOLESCENT MALE

CHIEF COMPLAINT

"Swelling around eyes and ankles."

HISTORY OF PRESENT ILLNESS

A 16-year-old boy of African-American and Filipino heritage arrives at his PCP office with his adoptive father for worsening swelling around his eyes and swollen ankles over the past week. He reports his eyes get puffy with seasonal allergies every fall, but they have never been this puffy. This morning, his feet were so swollen he could not put on shoes. He thought he had the stomach flu with loss of appetite, nausea, a couple of episodes of loose stool, and mild abdominal discomfort over the past week. He also states he has urinated only twice in the past 2 days. He has tried drinking more sports drink, but this has not helped. He works at a fast-food restaurant 3 evenings a week and admits French fries are a routine part of his diet. He plays on the school football team and has practice each day but wonders why he is so "out of shape" and exhausted. Today, he reports he is very tired, does not think he can participate in football practice, and is concerned his feet are too swollen for his cleats to fit.

REVIEW OF SYSTEMS

The patient's ROS is positive for loss of appetite, mild gastrointestinal upset, nausea, loose stool, reduced urinary output, and significant swelling of eyelids and lips, torso, legs, and feet over the past couple of days. He also reports fatigue, poor exercise tolerance, and mild SOB over the past week. The ROS is negative for fever, chills, rashes, vomiting, constipation, dysuria, hematuria, sore throat, cough, chest pain, backache, injuries, or trauma.

RELEVANT HISTORY

The patient's history is limited due to adoption at age 3. His adoptive father reports typical childhood illnesses since his adoption, with eczema as a toddler and seasonal allergies since age 9. He has asthma with URIs and exercise-induced asthma, onset 1 year ago. No known illness or injuries are reported. He was seen for a sports clearance exam with this provider 9 weeks ago. He measured 157.48 cm (62 in.) and weighed 51.25 kg (113 lbs). At that visit, urine dip was normal with only trace protein.

Before he was adopted, he was in foster care with an older sister for 2 years due to parental substance abuse. Perinatal drug exposure was suspected. His older biologic sister was adopted into another family and has a history of kidney transplant for unknown cause. He has no contact with his biologic parents or relatives. Adoptive parents have contact with the adoption agency and will seek more information about family and sibling medical history.

ALLERGIES

No known drug allergies; no known food allergies.

MEDICATIONS

- Albuterol HFA inhaler, 2 puffs 15 min pre-exercise and q4h PRN for asthma.
- Naproxen sodium 220 mg PO, occasional use for post-sports-activity muscle aches.

Physical Examination

Vitals: T 37°C (98.6°F), P 110, R 14, BP 122/62, SpO$_2$ 98%, HT 157.48 cm (62 in.), WT 55.79 kg (123 lbs), BMI 22.5. Note: 10 lbs weight gain from exam 9 weeks prior.

General: Mildly ill-appearing child alert and cooperative but with low energy.

Psychiatric: Fatigued, mildly anxious, but nondepressed appearing.

Skin, Hair, and Nails: Warm, dry, intact without rash; mild generalized swelling of trunk; mild edema of arms, moderate 3+ pitting edema lower extremities, especially ankles and feet, with moderate swelling extending into the scrotum.

Eyes: PERRLA; eyes are narrowed to slits due to periorbital edema.

ENT/Mouth: No lesions, posterior pharynx without erythema or exudate, uvula midline.

Neck: No cervical lymphadenopathy, no jugular venous distention, mild generalized edema of face and neck.

Lungs: Clear to auscultation bilaterally.

Heart: RRR; S1, S2 without murmur, gallop, or bruit.

Abdomen: Mild distention with generalized edema, non-tender, no hepatosplenomegaly, no costovertebral angle tenderness.

Genital/Rectal: Generalized swelling into scrotum; no testicular lesions, warmth, redness, tenderness, or masses; no penile discharge. Rectal exam was deferred.

Neurologic: A&O×3. Cranial nerves II to XII grossly intact, appropriate verbal responses.

Office-Based Lab: Urine dip SG 1.035, 3+ protein; negative glucose, blood, leukocytes, or nitrites. Note: urine dip on prior visit normal with only trace protein.

Clinical Discussion Question

1. What is the differential diagnosis?

_____

_____

_____

_____

2. What is the most likely diagnosis? Why?

_____

_____

_____

_____

3. Demonstrate your understanding about the pathophysiology in regard to the most likely diagnosis.

_____

_____

_____

_____

4. Should tests/imaging studies be ordered? Which ones? Why? Think about tests/imaging beyond the primary care setting as well.

_____

_____

_____

_____

5. What are the next appropriate steps in management?

_____

_____

_____

_____

6. Review a reliable, recent reference and demonstrate an understanding of the initial and long-term management of this diagnosis. Provide references for your response.

_____

_____

_____

_____

7. What are the pertinent ICD-10 and CPT (E/M) codes for this visit? Provide a short rationale.

_____

_____

_____

_____

8. What are appropriate patient and parent education topics for this case?

_____

_____

_____

_____

9. If not managed appropriately, what is/are the medical/legal concern(s) that may arise?

_____

_____

_____

_____

10. Think about interprofessional collaboration for this case. Provide a list of specialties or other disciplines and indicate what contribution these professionals might make to managing the patient.

_____

_____

_____

_____

BEDSIDE MANNER QUESTIONS

11. What would your communication style/approach be with this patient and adoptive father?

_____

_____

_____

_____

12. If a patient and his adoptive father are distressed by the diagnosis, what might offer support?

_____

_____

_____

_____

ANSWER KEY _available at_
https://connect.springerpub.com/content/book/978-0-8261-8273-9

BILATERAL HEEL PAIN, ADULT FEMALE

CHIEF COMPLAINT

"Bilateral heel pain."

HISTORY OF PRESENT ILLNESS

A 28-year-old obese woman presents as a new patient with a several-month history of bilateral heel pain. She denies any precipitating event, trauma, or specific incident that triggered her pain. The patient describes the heel pain as a sharp and stabbing sensation, exacerbated by prolonged standing and walking. The patient reports that the heel pain begins after taking the first few steps after getting out of bed.

She did go and see a local urgent care provider, who diagnosed the patient with overuse syndrome and prescribed ibuprofen, rest, and OTC inserts for her shoes. However, the patient reported minimal relief in her symptoms. She works as a grocery clerk and is on her feet 8 hours a day.

REVIEW OF SYSTEMS

The patient's ROS is positive for heel pain with prolonged standing and walking. Additionally, there is also pain at night. The patient's ROS is negative for bilateral swelling of the ankle, foot, and digits. She denies any altered sensation or weakness in both extremities. She also denies any gait abnormalities or flat feet, any temperature changes, any recent illnesses, or hospitalizations.

RELEVANT HISTORY

The patient's medical history is unremarkable other than obesity. She works in a local grocery as a grocery clerk. She is single and currently not sexually active. She doesn't drink alcohol or use any recreational drugs, and her family history is noncontributory.

MEDICATIONS

Ibuprofen 200 mg 1 or 2 tablets q6h PRN for pain.

ALLERGIES

No known drug allergies; no known food allergies.

PHYSICAL EXAMINATION

Vitals: T 37°C (98.6°F), P 84, R 20, BP 134/88, HT 167.6 cm (66 in.), WT 112.5 kg. (248 lbs), BMI 40.

General: No apparent distress.

Musculoskeletal/Bilateral Foot and Ankle: There is no swelling, deformity, crepitus, or bogginess of the feet and ankle. There are no skin changes. There is no tenderness over the forefoot and midfoot foot. ROM is as follows: dorsiflexion: 15/15, plantar flexion: 40/40, eversion: 20/20, inversion: 35/35, all without pain or discomfort. An anterior drawer test is negative. There is no lateral ligamentous laxity. There is mild hallux valgus deformity to both the great toes without tenderness. There is a negative Tinel's over the tibial and sural nerves. There is moderate pes cavus of both feet. There is no forefoot varus or "too many toes sign." There is no hindfoot valgus. There is no tenderness over the subtalar joint. There is exquisite point tenderness over the medial aspect of the calcaneal tuberosity. Heels are symmetrical without any bony masses palpated. Dorsalis pedis and posterior tibialis are 2+. Capillary refill is less than 2 seconds.

Neurologic: Sensation intact to the dorsal and plantar aspects of the foot, ankle, and leg. No signs of foot drop. No altered sensation compared to the contralateral extremity. No ankle clonus. Achilles reflex 2+.

CLINICAL DISCUSSION QUESTIONS

1. What is the differential diagnosis?

_____

_____

_____

_____

2. What is the most likely diagnosis? Why?

_____

_____

_____

_____

3. Demonstrate your understanding about the pathophysiology in regard to the most likely diagnosis.

_____

_____

_____

_____

4. Should tests/imaging studies be ordered? Which ones? Why? Think about tests/imaging beyond the primary care setting as well.

_____

_____

_____

_____

5. What are the next appropriate steps in management?

_____

_____

_____

6. Review a reliable, recent reference and demonstrate an understanding of the treatment recommendations associated with this diagnosis. Include the name of the references.

_____

_____

_____

_____

7. What are the pertinent ICD-10 and CPT (E/M) codes for this visit? Provide a short rationale.

_____

_____

_____

_____

8. What is the appropriate patient education for this case?

_____

_____

_____

_____

9. If not managed appropriately, what is/are the medical/legal concern(s) that may arise?

_____

_____

_____

_____

10. Think about interprofessional collaboration for this case. Provide a list of specialties or other disciplines and indicate what contribution these professionals might make to managing the patient.

_____

_____

_____

_____

Bedside Manner Question

11. What would your communication style/approach be with this patient?

_____

_____

_____

_____

Answer Key *available at*
https://connect.springerpub.com/content/book/978-0-8261-8273-9

DRY, CRACKED SKIN, ADULT FEMALE

CHIEF COMPLAINT

"Dry, cracked skin."

HISTORY OF PRESENT ILLNESS

A 32-year-old woman presents to her PCP with complaints of a persistent "scaly dry rash" just beneath the left knee. She states the condition is chronic, and it seems a little larger now and it has become bothersome at times. The condition is intermittent, itchy, and red. This time, she attempted to scratch it off but it started to hurt and bled when she "peeled" a little off. The patient then attempted OTC hydrocortisone cream and warm compresses, with some relief. Regardless of what she does, the rash comes back on the same spot. The patient explains that she is simply wanting better relief and answers. She thinks the scaly patch was worse during the winter months but is unsure. She has no history of allergies and has not changed soaps or daily routine. She has not been around anyone with any dermatologic conditions and reports no concerns with STIs.

REVIEW OF SYSTEMS

The patient's ROS is positive for increased stress, dry rash that is itchy and scaly, and increasing severity during winter months. Her ROS is negative for fever, nausea/vomiting, diarrhea, sore throat, other rashes, or sudden weight changes. She denies any exudates or blistering. The ROS is negative for angina and SOB.

RELEVANT HISTORY

The patient has a history of elevated BP and obesity. She is a full-time student and mother and works part-time in retail. She states her life stressors have been particularly difficult over the past year, including stress in her marriage. She has two children. She denies tobacco or drug use; she drinks socially. There is no family history of dermatologic or autoimmune conditions. Her family history is noncontributory.

ALLERGIES

No known drug allergies; no known food allergies.

MEDICATIONS

Ibuprofen 400 mg PRN TID for pain/bleed associated with rash.

PHYSICAL EXAMINATION

Vitals: T 37.2°C (98.9°F), P 82, R 19, BP 132/88, HT 170.2 cm (67 in.), WT 87.1 kg (192 lbs), BMI 32.

General: Alert; appears well hydrated and nourished and in no apparent distress.

Psychiatric: A&O with cognitive function being intact, cooperative with exam, good eye contact, and good insight.

Skin, Hair, and Nails: Patient has a scaly whitish-gray rash just inferior to the left patella, which appears as plaque. Some mild blood spots/pinpoints (possible Auspitz sign) noted. There is erythema noted throughout rash. Lichenification questionable. Hair and nails non-concerning.

Neck: Supple, FROM, no lymphadenopathy.

Chest: Normal chest rise/fall.

Lungs: Clear to auscultation bilaterally; no wheezes, rales, or rhonchi noted.

Heart: Normal sinus, no murmurs, normal rate, no jugular venous distention.

CLINICAL DISCUSSION QUESTIONS

1. What is the differential diagnosis?

_____

_____

_____

_____

2. What is the most likely diagnosis? Why?

_____

_____

_____

_____

3. Demonstrate your understanding about the pathophysiology in regard to the most likely diagnosis.

_____

_____

_____

_____

4. Should tests/imaging studies be ordered? Which ones? Why? Think about tests/imaging beyond the primary care setting as well.

_____

_____

_____

_____

5. What are the next appropriate steps in management?

_____

_____

_____

_____

6. Review a reliable, recent reference and discuss treatment approaches and comorbidities associated with this case. Provide the name of the references.

_____

_____

_____

_____

7. What are the pertinent ICD-10 and CPT (E/M) codes for this visit? Provide a short rationale.

_____

_____

_____

_____

8. What is the appropriate patient education for this case?

_____

_____

_____

_____

9. If not managed appropriately, what is/are the medical/legal concern(s) that may arise?

_____

_____

_____

_____

10. Think about interprofessional collaboration for this case. Provide a list of specialties or other disciplines and indicate what contribution these professionals might make to managing the patient.

_____

_____

_____

_____

Bedside Manner Question

11. What would your communication style/approach be with this patient?

_____

_____

_____

_____

Answer Key *available at*
https://connect.springerpub.com/content/book/978-0-8261-8273-9

URINE LEAKAGE, GERIATRIC FEMALE

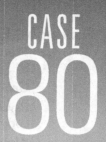

CASE
80

CHIEF COMPLAINT
"Urine leakage."

HISTORY OF PRESENT ILLNESS
A 66-year-old Caucasian woman presents with complaints of "leaking urine" and urgency of urination for 6 to 12 months. These symptoms have persisted to the point that she knows every public bathroom between her home and work and developed clear preferences for bathrooms in certain gas stations and fast food establishments. When she enters a new restaurant, she instinctively looks for the bathroom before being seated. Her concern is that when she is struck with the urge to urinate, she begins to leak, and she may not have more than a minute to get to the bathroom before she has an "accident." She experiences urinary frequency 8 to 10 times daily, often with episodes of leaking and occasionally with nocturia. She rates the symptoms as 7 of 10 on a bother scale.

Pelvic floor–strengthening exercises (Kegel exercises) and OTC herbal remedies have not helped. She experiences limited benefit from fluid restriction and is careful to urinate at home before driving. She wears pads to avoid the embarrassment of leaking and soiling her clothes in public.

REVIEW OF SYSTEMS
A ROS is positive for fatigue, nausea, abdominal pain, and hematuria. The patient reported headache and dizziness. The ROS is negative for fever, chills, glaucoma, vomiting, diarrhea, constipation, SOB, or chest pain.

RELEVANT HISTORY
Medical history is significant for Cesarean section (age 34) and a total hysterectomy (age 51) for menorrhagia. Her social history includes drinking 1 glass of wine per week since age 20, and she does not use recreational drugs. She admits to smoking a half pack of cigarettes per day for the last 10 years. Her two children are grown and have families of their own. She has suffered from intermittent depression since her husband died 8 years ago. Her family history is unremarkable.

ALLERGIES
No known drug allergies; no known food allergies.

MEDICATIONS
- Acetaminophen 500 mg PRN for arthralgia.
- Magnesium 250 mg nightly for sleep.
- Calcium 1,200 mg daily.
- Vitamin D 600 IU daily.
- Multivitamin daily.

Physical Examination

Vitals: T 36.9°C (98.4°F), P 76, R 14, BP 122/78, HT 168 cm (66 in.), WT 86 kg (189.5 lbs), BMI 30.5.

General: Well-developed, well-nourished, obese woman in no acute distress.

Psychiatric: Judgment and insight intact; rate of thoughts normal and logical; pleasant, calm, and cooperative; patient appears to be happy and content without overt anxiety or depression.

Abdomen: Active bowel sounds; abdomen soft, non-tender; no masses, no hernias, no suprapubic distension.

Genital/Rectal: No bladder tenderness on palpation and no distention noted. Atrophic external genitalia without prolapse, pelvic masses, or gross lesions. Vagina mucosa exhibits thinning and pallor with loss of rugae. No urinary leakage on cough test with a full bladder. On the rectal exam, perineal sensation intact; sphincter tone intact; able to contract the anal sphincter.

Neurologic: A&O×3; cranial nerves grossly intact; communication ability within normal limits; attention and concentration normal; sensation to light touch is intact; gait is within normal limits for age.

Clinical Discussion Questions

1. What is the differential diagnosis?

_____

_____

_____

2. What is the most likely diagnosis? Why?

_____

_____

_____

3. Demonstrate your understanding of the pathophysiology in regard to the most likely diagnosis.

_____

_____

_____

_____

4. Should tests/imaging studies be ordered? Which ones? Why? Think about tests/imaging beyond the primary care setting as well.

_____

_____

_____

_____

5. What are the next appropriate steps in management?

_____

_____

_____

_____

6. Review recent and credible research article(s) on this diagnosis. What are the helpful tools for making the diagnosis and treatment options? List your reference(s).

_____

_____

_____

_____

7. What are the pertinent ICD-10 and CPT (E/M) codes for this visit? Provide a short rationale.

_____

_____

_____

_____

8. What is the appropriate patient education topic for this case?

_____

_____

_____

_____

9. If not managed appropriately, what is/are the medical/legal concern(s) that may arise?

_____

_____

_____

_____

10. Think about interprofessional collaboration for this case. Provide a list of specialties or other disciplines and indicate what contribution these professionals might make to managing the patient.

_____

_____

_____

_____

BEDSIDE MANNER QUESTION

11. What would your communication style/approach be with this patient?

_____

_____

_____

_____

COUGHING AND GAGGING, PEDIATRIC MALE

CHIEF COMPLAINT
"Coughing and gagging."

HISTORY OF PRESENT ILLNESS

A mother brings her 3-month-old previously healthy infant to his PCP for evaluation of an apparent apnea episode that occurred that morning. He had developed a cough and nasal congestion about 5 days prior to this visit, and on the morning of the visit had a prolonged coughing spell followed by a gagging episode. His mother heard the cough and gagging over the baby monitor and when the gagging began, she ran to his room to check on him. By the time she picked him up from his crib, he did not seem to be breathing and his face and lips were blue. She immediately brought the baby to her husband, by which time the child had begun to breathe, and his color quickly returned to normal.

The episodes of cough have become more frequent and prolonged since the onset of the illness, but he has not had a fever. His mother reported she had been fighting off a "nagging cough" for about 3 weeks. The infant's 2-year-old sister and 4-year-old brother had no respiratory symptoms. None of the children attended day care.

REVIEW OF SYSTEMS

The infant's ROS is positive for decreased feeding and a few episodes of vomiting following coughing spells. The ROS is negative for fever, conjunctivitis, diarrhea, rash, or seizures.

RELEVANT HISTORY

The infant was born by vaginal delivery at 39 weeks' gestation following an uncomplicated pregnancy. His mother received regular prenatal care and had no history of untreated cervical infection. His birth weight was 6 lbs 14 oz, and he was discharged home at 48 hours of age after an uneventful stay in the newborn nursery. He had an appropriate weight gain and normal development and physical examination at his 2-week, 1-month, and 2-month well baby visits, and his routine newborn screening was normal. He had received all recommended immunizations, including those routinely administered at 2 months.

ALLERGIES

No known drug allergies; no known food allergies.

MEDICATIONS

None.

PHYSICAL EXAMINATION

Vitals: T 37.1°C (98.8°F); P 140; R 40; BP 80/40; SpO$_2$ 96%; HT 61 cm (24 in.), 43rd percentile; WT 5.5 kg (12 lbs), 10th percentile; BMI 14.6.

General: Alert and active, in no distress.

Skin, Hair, and Nails: Acyanotic, no rash or lesions. No abnormal findings with hair or nails.

Head: Anterior fontanelle soft and flat.

Eyes: No discharge or conjunctival injection.

ENT/Mouth: Nares congested, tympanic membranes clear, oral mucosa moist and without lesions.

Lungs: Clear to auscultation bilaterally, breath sounds equal bilaterally; no grunting, retractions, or nasal flaring.

Heart: RRR, S1 and S2 normal intensity, no murmur, pulses 2+ in all extremities.

Abdomen: Soft, no masses or hepatosplenomegaly.

Neurologic: Alert, moving all extremities equally, normal muscle bulk and tone.

CLINICAL DISCUSSION QUESTIONS

1. What is the differential diagnosis?

_____

_____

_____

_____

2. What is the most likely diagnosis? Why?

_____

_____

_____

_____

3. Demonstrate your understanding about the pathophysiology in regard to the most likely diagnosis.

_____

_____

_____

_____

4. Should tests/imaging studies be ordered? Which ones? Why? Think about tests/imaging beyond the primary care setting as well.

_____

_____

_____

_____

5. What are the next appropriate steps in management?

_____

_____

_____

_____

6. What are the preventive plans and treatment approaches for the diagnosis? Provide references for your response.

_____

_____

_____

_____

_____

7. What are the pertinent ICD-10 and CPT (E/M) codes for this visit? Provide a short rationale.

_____

_____

_____

_____

_____

8. What are appropriate parent education topics for this case?

_____

_____

_____

_____

9. If not managed appropriately, what is/are the medical/legal concern(s) that may arise?

_____

_____

_____

_____

10. Think about interprofessional collaboration for this case. Provide a list of specialties or other disciplines and indicate what contribution these professionals might make to managing the patient.

_____

_____

_____

_____

BEDSIDE MANNER QUESTIONS

11. What would your communication style/approach be with this patient's mother?

_____

_____

_____

_____

12. If the patient's mother is distressed by the diagnosis, what might offer support?

_____

_____

_____

_____

ANSWER KEY _available at_
https://connect.springerpub.com/content/book/978-0-8261-8273-9

EYE INJURY, ADULT MALE

CHIEF COMPLAINT
"Eye injury."

HISTORY OF PRESENT ILLNESS
A 32-year-old man presents to the clinic complaining of getting something in his left eye that he feels is still there. Just prior to presenting, he was stretching a bungee cord across the top of his kayak to secure it to the roof racks of his car, when the bungee cord snapped in half, ricocheting the rubber cord with the metal S hook toward his face. He reports something hitting his left eye as he could not get out of the way fast enough, has tried looking in a mirror to see if he could see what was in his eye, and has tried to flush out whatever might be stuck in his eye using all 16 oz of his bottled water. He reports the left eye pain as 10/10, stinging, sharp, throbbing, and very sensitive to light. He complains also of very blurry vision in the left eye, not being able to make much out, including shapes. He denies double vision, denies any eye injury in the past, does not wear corrective lenses of any kind, has not had eye surgery, and cannot recall his last tetanus immunization. He has not taken anything to alleviate the pain other than to hold an ice pack over his left eye. He denies any other injury to his face, mouth, or teeth. He is here with his wife.

REVIEW OF SYSTEMS
The patient's ROS is positive for foreign body sensation in the left eye with severe pain, photosensitivity, excessive tearing, redness and extreme blurred vision in left eye, and throbbing headache behind left eye. His ROS is negative for double vision, spots, specks, flashing lights, corrective lenses, facial lacerations, abrasions, or head injury.

RELEVANT HISTORY
The patient has no contributory medical or surgical history. He is happily married and father of two children. He is a social drinker. He denies tobacco or drug use. His family history is noncontributory.

ALLERGIES
Sulfonamides create rash and intense pruritis; no known food allergies.

MEDICATIONS
Multivitamin PO daily.

PHYSICAL EXAMINATION
Vitals: T 37.2°C (99.0°F), P 114, R 16, BP 148/94, HT 185.4 cm (73 in.), WT 86.2 kg (190 lbs), BMI 25.1.

General: Frightened male of stated age, worried about left eye vision. A&O; answers all questions appropriately.

Skin, Hair, and Nails: Warm throughout; no lesions, lacerations, ecchymosis. No abnormal findings with hair or nails.

Head: Atraumatic, normocephalic, non-tender.

Eyes: No periorbital lacerations, lesions, ecchymosis, step offs, or tenderness bilaterally.

Left eye: Swollen and tender upper and lower lids, good position, unable to close fully. Injected sclera and hyperemic conjunctiva, subconjunctival hemorrhage at the medial canthus extending to the iris, excessive tearing, tear-drop-shaped pupil not reactive to light or accommodation. Foreign body not visible to the naked eye. No fluid visualized as being emitted from the anterior or lateral portions of the globe. EOMs limited in movement. Difficult to assess retinal structures funduscopically due to patient's pain level and difficulty with visualization.

Right eye: No lid edema, good position and closure, injected sclera, pink conjunctive. Pupil 4 mm, round, reactive to light and accommodation. EOMIs intact, no disc edema or swelling, venous pulsations, or AV nicking.

ENT/Mouth: Hearing acuity intact bilaterally to whispered voice. No deformities, lacerations, lesions, or tenderness externally, bilaterally. TMs pearly gray, positive cone of light; no discharge or bleeding bilaterally. No maxillary or frontal sinus tenderness. Nares patent, septum midline, dark pink mucosa with clear nasal drainage L>R. Teeth and gums in good repair; no bleeding. Oral mucosa and tongue without lesions or lacerations, oropharynx patent, tonsils 1+ and symmetric, uvula midline.

Neck: FROM, supple, no adenopathy.

Neurologic: Cranial nerve II grossly intact OD; unable to assess cranial nerve II OS due to extreme blurred vision. Cranial nerves III to XII grossly intact.

CLINICAL DISCUSSION QUESTIONS

1. What is the differential diagnosis?

_____

_____

_____

_____

2. What is the most likely diagnosis? Why?

_____

_____

_____

_____

3. Demonstrate your understanding about the pathophysiology in regard to the most likely diagnosis.

_____

_____

_____

_____

4. Should tests/imaging studies be ordered? Which ones? Why? Think about tests/imaging beyond the primary care setting as well.

_____

_____

_____

_____

_____

5. What are the next appropriate steps in management?

_____

_____

_____

_____

_____

6. What are the treatment approaches, prevalence, and physical exam techniques of this diagnosis? Provide references for your responses.

_____

_____

_____

_____

_____

7. What are the pertinent ICD-10 and CPT (E/M) codes for this visit? Provide a short rationale.

_____

_____

_____

_____

_____

8. What are the appropriate patient education topics for this case?

_____

_____

_____

_____

_____

9. If not managed appropriately, what is/are the medical/legal concern(s) that may arise?

_____

_____

_____

_____

_____

10. Think about interprofessional collaboration for this case. Provide a list of specialties or other disciplines and indicate what contribution these professionals might make to managing the patient.

_____

_____

_____

_____

_____

BEDSIDE MANNER QUESTIONS

11. What would your communication style/approach be with this patient and his wife?

_____

_____

_____

_____

_____

12. If a patient and his wife are distressed by the diagnosis, what might offer support?

_____

_____

_____

_____

_____

ANSWER KEY _available at_
https://connect.springerpub.com/content/book/978-0-8261-8273-9

PAIN IN GREAT TOE, ADULT FEMALE

CHIEF COMPLAINT

"Pain in great toe."

HISTORY OF PRESENT ILLNESS

A 54-year-old woman presents with complaints of right great toe pain that has been bothering her for the past 4 to 6 weeks. She states the pain has been a constant 5/10 and is somewhat relieved with ibuprofen and changing positions frequently. She cannot recall what caused this pain, denying any trauma to the toe or foot. A few weeks ago, the pain became so annoying she sought medical attention in an ED. She reports she underwent x-rays of her right foot and great toe, both of which were negative for fracture. She states she was told that a fracture may not show up on film right away, so she would need to follow up with an orthopedic specialist within 2 weeks to obtain new x-rays. The ED provider buddy-taped her right great toe to the adjacent toe, placed her in a post-op shoe, and asked her to limit weight bearing and to continue to take ibuprofen for pain.

She denies arthritis, gout, blood clots, and previous injury/trauma to her right foot or great toe. She denies radiation of the pain into her calf but does admit there are times when she feels her right great toe goes numb. The pain returns when she stands up from a sitting position, stands for prolonged periods of time, climbs stairs, sits on a hard chair, or drives a car. She admits to being in a car accident 3 months ago, where she was the driver who was rear-ended at a stop light. She refused to be taken to the ED at that time, complaining only of minimal neck pain, which has resolved. She states she has experienced low back spasms that come and go since then and denies any diagnostic studies of her lower spine.

REVIEW OF SYSTEMS

The patient's ROS is positive for pain in the right great toe and lower back spasms. Her ROS is negative for fever, chills, diaphoresis, insomnia, urinary problems, bowel movement changes, or recent unintentional weight loss or gain. The patient denies rashes, lumps, lesions, itchiness, dryness, color changes, or change in nails or hair. She also denies swollen glands, pain or stiffness, leg cramps, varicose veins, or history of DVT.

RELEVANT HISTORY

The patient has a history of hypertension, hypercholesterolemia, hypertriglyceridemia, and fibrocystic breast disease. She has a 20-pack-year tobacco history and quit 8 years ago. She drinks two glasses of red wine on the weekends and denies illicit or recreational drug use. Her diet is rich in seafood, especially shrimp and fish. She does not eat organ meats or consume caffeine. Her family history is significant for hypertension, type 2 diabetes, hypercholesterolemia, angina, and glaucoma.

ALLERGIES

No known drug allergies; no known food allergies.

MEDICATIONS

- Amlodipine 10 mg PO QD
- Chlorthalidone 25 mg PO QD
- Rosuvastatin 40 mg PO QD
- Ibuprofen 400 mg PO q6h PRN for right great toe pain.

PHYSICAL EXAMINATION

Vitals: T 37°C (98.6°F), P 80, R 14, BP 154/92, HT 168 cm (66 in.), WT 66.2 kg (146 lbs), BMI 23.6.

General: Pleasant female of stated age in no acute distress, sitting in chair adjacent to exam table. A&O.

Skin, Hair, and Nails: No erythema, rashes, lesions, or masses. No abnormal findings with hair or nails.

Neck: FROM, supple without tenderness.

Peripheral Vascular: Warm throughout, all pulses 2+ symmetric bilaterally, capillary refill < 2 seconds throughout.

Musculoskeletal: No curvatures of the spine, slight pelvic tilt with left iliac crest slightly higher than right. Tender L3 to L5 spinous processes without step-offs. Painful right-sided paravertebral muscle spasms initiated with deep palpation of L4 to L5 and right sciatic nerve within the right buttock with patient positioned in fetal position. Decreased ROM L-spine, right lateral bending. No deformities at BLEs; tender right first metatarsophalangeal joint without increased warmth, swelling, or erythema. FROM at left lower extremity. FROM at right lower extremity except decreased ROM at right great toe in flexion and extension.

Neurologic: Cranial nerves II to XII grossly intact; speech appropriate; antalgic gait favoring right foot. L1, L2, L3, S1, S2: sharp/dull discrimination and vibratory sense intact at BLEs L4, L5: sharp/dull discrimination and vibratory sense intact at left lower extremity. Unable to discriminate dull sensation, at lateral aspect of right calf, extending distally to right mid-foot and great toe.

CLINICAL DISCUSSION QUESTIONS

1. What is the differential diagnosis?

_____

_____

_____

_____

2. What is the most likely diagnosis? Why?

_____

_____

_____

_____

3. Demonstrate your understanding about the pathophysiology in regard to the most likely diagnosis.

_____

_____

_____

_____

4. Should tests/imaging studies be ordered? Which ones? Why? Think about tests/imaging beyond the primary care setting as well.

_____

_____

_____

_____

5. What are the next appropriate steps in management?

_____

_____

_____

_____

6. What is the treatment approach for this diagnosis? Provide your references(s).

_____

_____

_____

_____

7. What are the pertinent ICD-10 and CPT (E/M) codes for this visit? Provide a short rationale.

_____

_____

_____

_____

8. What is the appropriate patient education for this case?

_____

_____

_____

_____

9. If not managed appropriately, what is/are the medical/legal concern(s) that may arise?

_____

_____

_____

_____

10. Think about interprofessional collaboration for this case. Provide a list of specialties or other disciplines and indicate what contribution these professionals might make to managing the patient.

_____

_____

_____

_____

BEDSIDE MANNER QUESTION

11. What would your communication style/approach be with this patient?

_____

_____

_____

_____

ANSWER KEY available at
https://connect.springerpub.com/content/book/978-0-8261-8273-9

BILATERAL LEG PAIN, PEDIATRIC MALE

CHIEF COMPLAINT
"Bilateral leg pain."

HISTORY OF PRESENT ILLNESS
A woman brings in her 5-year-old African American son for an evaluation of worsening leg pain over the past 2 days. She states the boy started complaining of leg pain in both legs 2 days ago, after waking in the morning. She denies any known provoking trauma or falls and has not seen any evidence of injury to his legs. The boy points to both of his legs and states the pain is "all over inside." The boy's mother denies noticing any swelling or bruising of the legs and denies the boy having any similar symptoms in the past. The mother states her son is usually very active but has not been able to play or run due to the pain. The boy is crying due to pain, which prompted her to come in for evaluation. The mother tried applying warm and cold packs to his legs, without relief. She gave the boy a dose of acetaminophen yesterday morning without relief; however, the dose of ibuprofen she gave this morning seemed to calm him down a little.

REVIEW OF SYSTEMS
The patient's ROS is positive for bilateral leg pain L = R, with gait disturbance due to pain. His ROS is negative for fever, chills, weakness, vomiting, change in bowel, cough, SOB, and history of joint or bone pain.

RELEVANT HISTORY
The child's history is significant for a full-term birth at 39 weeks, born in a small rural village in Martinique, at home, to his mother without pregnancy complications. His family immigrated to the United States when the patient was 3 years old. His immunizations are up to date. He has no history of neonatal infections or hospitalizations. He has met all developmental milestones, and growth trajectories are stable at 25th percentile for height and weight. He was diagnosed with strep throat last fall and treated with 7 days of antibiotics. He lives with his parents, attends pre-K full time, and eats a balanced diet. His mother is healthy, age 28 years. His father has an undiagnosed "blood condition" that caused him to be hospitalized for 3 days when he was 20 years old.

ALLERGIES
No known drug, food, or environmental allergies.

MEDICATIONS
None.

PHYSICAL EXAMINATION
Vitals: T 37°C (98.6°F); P 125; R 24; BP 98/54; HT 107 cm (42 in.), 25th percentile; WT 17 kg (37.4 lbs), 25th percentile; BMI 14.9. Growth on trajectory since initial visit at age 3 years.

General: Slender boy, laying on exam table in mild distress, whimpering in pain at times, nontoxic appearing.

Skin, Hair, Nails: No rashes, skin warm to touch with increased warmth of BLE compared to trunk/arms, full head of hair on scalp. No abnormal findings with nails.

Head: Normocephalic, atraumatic.

Eyes: Mild scleral icterus bilaterally, conjunctiva clear bilaterally.

ENT/Mouth: Oropharynx clear with 2+ tonsillar hypertrophy bilat; no erythema or exudates noted. Nares patent bilaterally without drainage. Normal dentition, gums pink and moist. Moist mucous membranes.

Neck: Supple, with shotty anterior bilateral cervical lymphadenopathy, non-tender.

Chest: No deformity.

Lungs: Clear to auscultation bilaterally without wheezes/ronchi/crackles.

Heart: RRR without murmur, prominent point of maximal impulse.

Abdomen: Soft, non-tender, non-distended, spleen tip palpable.

Genital/Rectal: Uncircumcised penis, Tanner stage 1.

Musculoskeletal: Normal bulk. Lower extremities without deformity or erythema. BLEs show increased warmth to palpation compared to trunk/upper extremities. Non-tender to palpation over bony prominences of lower extremities or knee/ankle joints. No edema or effusion noted bilaterally. Able to bear weight. Bilateral FROM lower extremities while supine. Strength 5/5 BLEs.

Neurologic: Alert, refusal to stand due to pain but cranial nerves II to XII intact. BLE DTRs 2+ intact.

CLINICAL DISCUSSION QUESTIONS

1. What is the differential diagnosis?

_____

_____

_____

_____

_____

2. What is the most likely diagnosis? Why?

_____

_____

_____

_____

_____

3. Demonstrate your understanding about the pathophysiology in regard to the most likely diagnosis.

_____

_____

_____

_____

4. Should tests/imaging studies be ordered? Which ones? Why? Think about tests/imaging beyond the primary care setting as well.

_____

_____

_____

_____

_____

5. What are the next appropriate steps in management?

_____

_____

_____

_____

_____

6. What are the risk factors, early symptoms, and treatment approach of the diagnosis? Provide references for your responses.

_____

_____

_____

_____

_____

7. What are the pertinent ICD-10 and CPT (E/M) codes for this visit? Provide a short rationale.

_____

_____

_____

_____

_____

8. What are appropriate parent/patient education topics for this case?

_____

_____

_____

_____

_____

9. If not managed appropriately, what is/are the medical/legal concern(s) that may arise?

_____

_____

_____

_____

_____

10. Think about interprofessional collaboration for this case. Provide a list of specialties or other disciplines and indicate what contribution these professionals might make to managing the patient.

_____

_____

_____

_____

_____

BEDSIDE MANNER QUESTIONS

11. What would your communication style/approach be with this parent and patient?

_____

_____

_____

_____

_____

12. If a patient and his mother are distressed by the diagnosis, what might offer support?

_____

_____

_____

_____

_____

ANSWER KEY _available at_
https://connect.springerpub.com/content/book/978-0-8261-8273-9

CONFUSION, GERIATRIC FEMALE

CHIEF COMPLAINT
"Confusion."

HISTORY OF PRESENT ILLNESS

An 80-year-old woman with mild Parkinson's disease, severe generalized anxiety disorder, gastroesophageal reflux disease, and chronic urinary retention with recurrent UTIs is brought in to her PCP's office by her daughter because of mild confusion over the past 2 days. The daughter has observed her compulsively taking her temperature and wandering around the house, repeatedly stating, "Am I septic?" The patient, who is typically sharp and lucid, called her PCP 2 weeks ago complaining of urinary urgency and incontinence but refused an office visit or urine test because she was "too busy" with other appointments. Considering her history and upon review of her most recent urine culture and sensitivity testing performed 2 months prior, a prescription for nitrofurantoin was called in to her pharmacy, she was given ED precautions, and she was advised to schedule a follow-up appointment in 1 week.

Today, the patient states she did not come in because her urinary symptoms improved, but she admits she feels worse overall, endorsing nausea, anorexia, weight loss, diffuse body aches, chills, and night sweats, which she attributes to her new medication for PD, which was started 6 months ago. She denies dysuria, hematuria, fever, or flank pain but notes she "never has" dysuria with her UTIs. "I just shiver when I get the enterococcus; that's how I know it's not the *E. coli*." She asks repeatedly "Do I have sepsis?" because home temperature "always runs 96.8," which is "too low" according to her internet research. She has not returned to her urologist in over a year. "He just wants to give me another pill; I won't take it."

The patient's daughter, who works two jobs and is not home much, states that the patient is not compliant with prescribed medications, even with a pill box. The patient carefully reads all pharmacy package inserts, gets scared by the lists of side effects, and then searches the internet to see how "dangerous" the medication is before deciding whether she will take it. The patient admits she cuts most pills in half or takes less than the prescribed dose because she is "allergic to everything." The patient states she only took the nitrofurantoin pill once a day instead of BID and for only 4 of the 7 days prescribed. "I hate that pill. I get so nauseated." She doesn't trust prescription medications in general. "I read the internet, I know about pharma, I want natural antibiotics, D-mannose, cranberry."

REVIEW OF SYSTEMS

The patient's ROS is positive for chills, weight loss, fatigue, constipation, rectal wipe-bleeding and rectal discomfort "when hemorrhoids swell," insomnia, depression, and anxiety. It is positive for vaginal itching and pain, chronic, without discharge or bleeding. It is positive for skin itching "all over" but no rash. Her ROS is negative for fever. She has no cough, SOB, or dyspnea on exertion. It is negative for chest pain, palpitations, dizziness, or edema; abdominal pain, vomiting, or melena; weakness, paresthesia, or dysarthria; or forgetfulness or getting lost.

RELEVANT HISTORY

In addition to PD, severe GAD, GERD, and chronic urinary retention/recurrent UTIs, the patient has essential hypertension, hyperlipidemia, impaired fasting glucose, gout, hypothyroidism, hearing loss (refuses hearing aids), and allergic rhinitis.

The patient underwent open cholecystectomy in 1967, thyroidectomy in 1978, and TAH/BSO in 1985, all for benign conditions. She absolutely refuses mammograms, colon cancer screening, and vaccinations, due to fear of side effects.

Her mother died at 71 from heart disease; her father died at 90 from "old age." Her brother died at 78 from prostate cancer, and one daughter, age 54, has bipolar disorder. The patient is a widow and retired high school teacher with a master's degree; she drinks one glass of wine once per week and has never smoked or used recreational drugs. She moved in with her daughter 10 years ago, when her husband died, and does not drive due to anxiety. She eats "whatever sounds good" and gets no exercise other than going to her appointments and has no outside interest or hobbies.

ALLERGIES

No known drug allergies; no known food allergies.

MEDICATIONS

- Prescribed medications include the following:
  - Levothyroxine 100 mcg QD
  - Allopurinol 100 mg QD
  - Metoprolol succinate ER 25 mg QD
  - Carbidopa-levodopa 25 mg/100 mg TID
  - Vitamin D 2000 IU QD
  - Polyethylene glycol 3350 17 g in 8 oz fluid QD
  - Loratadine 10 mg QD
  - Diazepam 2 mg BID PRN for anxiety/insomnia
- She has been using an expired prescription for triamcinolone acetonide 0.1% cream on her vulva BID for itching for the last 6 months.
- She continues to take conjugated estrogens 0.3 mg PO QD prescribed by her urologist.
- She has stopped all GERD medications because they give her a headache.

PHYSICAL EXAMINATION

Vitals: T 36.7°C (98.1°F), P 74, R 14, BP 132/60, SpO$_2$ 98%, HT 160 cm (63 in.), WT 89.8 kg. (198 lbs), BMI 35.1 (weight down 3 lbs in 5 months).

General: Well-developed, well-appearing, overnourished older female, A&O×3. All vital signs stable. In no acute distress; ate entire bag of chips and drank one can of a nutrition supplement during interview.

Psychiatric: Labile affect, pressured and tangential speech with logorrhea (no change from patient's baseline); fair insight.

Skin, Hair, and Nails: Warm and dry, no rashes noted on full skin exam. Moist, sticky intertriginous areas present in inframammary, intergluteal, and inguinal regions. No abnormal findings with hair or nails.

Lungs: Clear to auscultation bilaterally with no adventitious sounds noted.

Heart: RRR with no murmurs, gallops, or rubs.

Abdomen: Normoactive bowel sounds in four quadrants with no bruits noted. Soft, non-tender, non-distended; no masses, hepatosplenomegaly, or hernia present. Surgical scars at RUQ and midline lower are well healed. No costovertebral angle tenderness elicited.

Genital/Rectal: External genitalia, Bartholin glands, urethra, and Skene glands fully obscured by talcum powder; vaginal mucosa pink but extremely dry and thin with no abnormal discharge noted. Swab of vaginal vault obtained for wet mount. Tender anal canal with multiple moderate-sized non-thrombosed external and internal hemorrhoids and no fissures noted; tan soft stool in vault; heme negative.

Musculoskeletal: Good muscle tone; no clubbing or cyanosis; radial pulses 2+ bilaterally.

Neurologic: Slow but steady gait without shuffling; no tremors or cogwheeling noted; 5/5 strength BLEs with sensation intact to light touch bilaterally. Gross hearing decreased bilaterally. MMSE score 27/30.

CLINICAL DISCUSSION QUESTIONS

1. What is the differential diagnosis?

_____

_____

_____

_____

_____

2. What is the most likely diagnosis? Why?

_____

_____

_____

_____

_____

_____

3. Demonstrate your understanding about the pathophysiology in regard to the most likely diagnosis.

_____

_____

_____

_____

_____

4. Should tests/imaging studies be ordered? Which ones? Why? Think about tests/imaging beyond the primary care setting as well.

_____

_____

_____

_____

_____

5. What are the next appropriate steps in management?

_____

_____

_____

_____

_____

6. What is the clinical presentation of the older adult, and what is the initial treatment associated with the diagnosis? Provide references for your response.

_____

_____

_____

_____

_____

7. What are the pertinent ICD-10 and CPT (E/M) codes for this visit? Provide a short rationale.

_____

_____

_____

_____

_____

8. What are the appropriate patient education topics for this case?

_____

_____

_____

_____

_____

9. If not managed appropriately, what is/are the medical/legal concern(s) that may arise?

_____

_____

_____

_____

_____

10. Think about interprofessional collaboration for this case. Provide a list of specialties or other disciplines and indicate what contribution these professionals might make to managing the patient.

_____

_____

_____

_____

_____

BEDSIDE MANNER QUESTION

11. What would your communication style/approach be with this patient?

_____

_____

_____

_____

_____

_____

ANSWER KEY *available at*
https://connect.springerpub.com/content/book/978-0-8261-8273-9

LUMP IN THROAT, ADULT MALE

CHIEF COMPLAINT
"Lump in throat."

HISTORY OF PRESENT ILLNESS
A 35-year-old man arrives at his PCP's office reporting the sensation of a lump in his throat for over 1 month and episodes of mild epigastric pain with occasional nausea. He has experienced bloating and belching. He has a dry cough and feels like he needs to clear his throat often. He has a sour taste in his mouth and states that he frequently gets painful canker sores. He also complains of a burning type of pain to the anterior chest. The burning pain starts in the upper chest area and works its way up to the neck and throat area. He experiences the symptoms daily, and they become worse when he lies down or after eating.

REVIEW OF SYSTEMS
The patient's ROS is positive for nausea, bloating, belching, cough, canker sores, chest pain, and repetitive throat clearing. His ROS is negative for sore throat, hoarseness, dysphagia, vomiting, abdominal pain, melena, weight loss, change in appetite, asthma, ear pain, tooth pain, or exertional type chest pain. He denies a cardiac history or hypertension. He does not smoke. He occasionally drinks alcohol and daily drinks caffeinated soda. He denies any SOB or wheezing.

RELEVANT HISTORY
The patient has a history of Paget Schroetter syndrome at age 25. He is a full-time high school teacher. He exercises regularly. He is sexually active in a long-term relationship with his live-in girl-friend. His family history includes both grandparents with diabetes and hypertension. His father, who is living, has a history of stage 4 throat cancer at age 55.

ALLERGIES
No known drug allergies; no known food allergies.

MEDICATIONS
None.

PHYSICAL EXAMINATION
Vitals: T 37.2°C (98.8°F), P 82, R 20, BP 120/80, HT 193 cm (76 in.), WT 127 kg (280 lbs), BMI 34.08.

General: Alert and cooperative. Sitting comfortably on exam table. Well nourished. No acute distress.

Psychiatric: Mildly anxious.

ENT/Mouth: Tympanic membranes clear; canals clear bilaterally. Nose with no nasal septal deviation; mucous membranes moist and pink. Throat with pink and moist oropharynx; no erythema, no tonsillar enlargement, no lesions, no tooth erosion. Mouth with no sores or lesions present.

Neck: Supple with no lymphadenopathy; thyroid normal size.

Chest: Symmetric with no palpated tenderness.

Lungs: Clear to auscultation bilaterally; no rales, wheezes, or rhonchi.

Heart: RRR; no murmurs or gallops.

Abdomen: Non-distended and soft with normal active bowel sounds present in all quadrants; no pain on palpation of the abdomen.

CLINICAL DISCUSSION QUESTIONS

1. What is the differential diagnosis?

_____

_____

_____

2. What is the most likely diagnosis? Why?

_____

_____

_____

3. Demonstrate your understanding about the pathophysiology in regard to the most likely diagnosis.

_____

_____

_____

4. Should tests/imaging studies be ordered? Which ones? Why? Think about tests/imaging beyond the primary care setting as well.

_____

_____

_____

5. What are the next appropriate steps in management?

_____

_____

_____

_____

6. What is the prevalence and treatment approach of the diagnosis and the risks associated with the medications when used long term? Provide references(s) for your response.

_____

_____

_____

_____

7. What are the pertinent ICD-10 and CPT (E/M) codes for this visit? Provide a short rationale.

_____

_____

_____

_____

8. What is the appropriate patient education topic for this case?

_____

_____

_____

_____

9. If not managed appropriately, what is/are the medical/legal concern(s) that may arise?

_____

_____

_____

_____

10. Think about interprofessional collaboration for this case. Provide a list of specialties or other disciplines and indicate what contribution these professionals might make to managing the patient.

_____

_____

_____

_____

BEDSIDE MANNER QUESTION

11. What would your communication style/approach be with this patient?

_____

_____

_____

_____

ANSWER KEY *available at*
https://connect.springerpub.com/content/book/978-0-8261-8273-9

FEVER AND RASH, ADULT MALE

CHIEF COMPLAINT

"Fever and rash."

HISTORY OF PRESENT ILLNESS

A 22-year-old man presents to the office for the first time with an influenza-like illness he has had for the past week. Symptoms developed gradually and consist of fever (measured at home up to 101.4°F), sore throat, fatigue, anorexia, myalgias, and a mild diffuse headache. Yesterday, he noted an erythematous rash on the arms, torso, and legs, which prompted his visit today. He denies any known sick contacts, unusual exposures, or recent travel.

REVIEW OF SYSTEMS

The patient denies chills. He denies stiff neck or any focal neurologic complaints. He denies rhinorrhea, ear pain or discharge, sinus pressure or discharge, cough, SOB, chest pain, abdominal pain, nausea, vomiting, diarrhea, dysuria, hematuria, penile discharge, or arthralgia. A comprehensive ROS is otherwise unremarkable.

RELEVANT HISTORY

The patient has no history of significant medical problems or STIs. He has not had any recent dental procedures. Since last year he has been on HIV PrEP. He is currently taking tenofovir/emtricitabine. He tested negative for HIV about 10 weeks ago as it is a recommended screening every three months while on PrEP. He received a flu shot this past fall. He received meningococcal vaccination prior to entering college. He otherwise believes he is up to date on all required immunizations. The patient is a graduate student in civil engineering. He drinks alcohol at parties on weekends and has no history of tobacco use or vaping. He does not use any illicit substances, including marijuana. He is sexually active with men; he broke up with his previous partner 7 to 8 months ago, and he does not have a current partner. His last sexual activity was approximately 2 months ago after meeting someone at a party. The patient's family history is negative for chronic or recurrent infections; it has been reviewed and is otherwise noncontributory.

ALLERGIES

No known drug allergies; no known food allergies.

MEDICATIONS

Tenofovir/emtricitabine 25 mg/200 mg QD.

PHYSICAL EXAMINATION

Vitals: T 37.7°C (99.8°F), P 86, R 12, BP 125/80, HT 175 cm (69 in.), WT 70 kg (154 lbs), BMI 22.7.

General: Thin male in no acute distress.

Psychiatric: Normal mood and affect.

Skin, Hair, and Nails: Skin: There is a faint maculopapular rash on torso, back, and the upper and lower extremities including the palms and soles. No abnormal findings with hair or nails.

Head: Normocephalic, atraumatic.

Eyes: No scleral icterus.

ENT/Mouth: Sinuses non-tender to palpation. Poor dentition without gingival inflammation or tenderness to palpation. No foul odor to the breath.

Neck: Supple, FROM. No cervical lymphadenopathy.

Chest: Non-tender to palpation.

Lungs: Clear to auscultation bilaterally.

Heart: RRR without murmur.

Abdomen: Soft, non-tender, non-distended, active bowel sounds, no organomegaly, no masses felt.

Genital/Rectal: No lesions noted. No penile discharge. Scrotum non-tender. Multiple small, non-tender inguinal lymph nodes are palpable bilaterally. Rectal exam deferred.

Musculoskeletal: No inflammation or tenderness to palpation diffusely.

Neurologic: A&O×3, grossly non-focal.

CLINICAL DISCUSSION QUESTIONS

1. What is the differential diagnosis?

_____

_____

_____

_____

2. What is the most likely diagnosis? Why?

_____

_____

_____

_____

3. Demonstrate your understanding about the pathophysiology in regard to the most likely diagnosis.

_____

_____

_____

_____

_____

4. Should tests/imaging studies be ordered? Which ones? Why? Think about tests/imaging beyond the primary care setting as well.

_____

_____

_____

_____

_____

5. What are the next appropriate steps in management?

_____

_____

_____

_____

_____

6. What is the level of understanding of this diagnosis among noninfectious disease providers? What is the treatment recommendation for this diagnosis? List the references you consulted.

_____

_____

_____

_____

_____

7. What are the pertinent ICD-10 and CPT (E/M) codes for this visit? Provide a short rationale.

_____

_____

_____

_____

8. What is the appropriate patient education for this case?

_____

_____

_____

_____

9. If not managed appropriately, what is/are the medical/legal concern(s) that may arise?

_____

_____

_____

_____

_____

10. Think about interprofessional collaboration for this case. Provide a list of specialties or other disciplines and indicate what contribution these professionals might make to managing the patient.

_____

_____

_____

_____

_____

_____

BEDSIDE MANNER QUESTIONS

11. What would your communication style/approach be with this patient?

_____

_____

_____

_____

_____

12. If a patient is distressed by the diagnosis, what might offer support?

_____

_____

_____

_____

_____

ANSWER KEY *available at*
https://connect.springerpub.com/content/book/978-0-8261-8273-9

EXTREME WEAKNESS, ADULT MALE

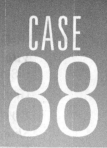

CHIEF COMPLAINT

"Extreme weakness."

HISTORY OF PRESENT ILLNESS

A 22-year-old Vietnamese male was carried into his PCP's office by two male family members. The family members told the nurse the patient is weak and unable to walk on his own. The patient had immigrated to the United States from Vietnam 2 years ago and has no previously diagnosed major medical problems. His weakness started yesterday, initially as muscle cramps, which gradually progressed to generalized muscle weakness. He denied any muscle pain and has had no associated symptoms. He denied any injury and any psychiatric problems. The patient mentioned that the weakness started in his lower extremities first and then gradually progressed to his upper extremities. He denied any breathing problems. The patient also stated that he was at a birthday party the day before his symptoms started and he ate a large meal containing rice.

REVIEW OF SYSTEMS

The patient's ROS is positive for generalized muscle weakness, fatigue, and muscle cramps; he is unable to walk. His ROS is negative for any recent weight loss, fever, chills, nausea, vomiting, headaches or URI symptoms, SOB, chest pain, or abdominal pain. The review is also negative for any urinary symptoms or mood changes or depression.

RELEVANT HISTORY

The patient is Vietnamese and has only been in the United States a few years. He has occasional mild seasonal asthma. He smokes half a pack of cigarettes a day. Once a week, he has one or two beers. He denies any THC or illicit drug use. He lives with his older brother in an apartment. He works as a store clerk at a convenience store and has no unusual stress at work. He has no girlfriend at this time and has not been sexually active for a few months. His father had a heart attack at age 50; his mother is healthy. Both live in Vietnam. His older brother had been hospitalized for an unknown medical condition.

ALLERGIES

No known drug or food allergies.

MEDICATIONS

None.

PHYSICAL EXAMINATION

Vitals: T 98.2°F (36.8°C), BP 128/74, P 110, R 12, SPO$_2$ 98%, WT 72.57 kg (160 lbs), HT 172.7 cm (68 in.), BMI 24.3.

General: Appeared anxious and weak but in no other distress. Nontoxic.

Psychiatric: Normal mood and affect.

Skin, Hair, and Nails: Clear with no rashes, lesions, or petechiae or purpura. No abnormal findings with hair or nails.

ENT/Mouth: TM clear bilaterally, no discharge in the ears, oral mucosa moist, no pharyngeal erythema.

Neck: Soft and supple with no nuchal rigidity or thyromegaly.

Chest: Adequate and symmetric chest expansion.

Lungs: Clear bilaterally with no wheezing, rales, or rhonchi.

Heart: Mild tachycardia but regular with no murmurs or gallops.

Abdomen: Soft. Non-tender. No palpable masses or organomegaly. Bowel sounds normal.

Lymphatic: No palpable lymphadenopathy symmetrically.

Musculoskeletal: Patient had diffuse muscle weakness at 2/5 of all his large muscle groups in all extremities. No muscle tenderness. He was unable to walk due to generalized weakness.

Neurologic: A&O×3. Cranial nerves II to XII grossly normal. No detectable sensory deficits. DTRs 1+ bilaterally; decreased symmetrically.

CLINICAL DISCUSSION QUESTIONS

1. What is the differential diagnosis?

_____

_____

_____

_____

_____

2. What is the most likely diagnosis? Why?

_____

_____

_____

_____

_____

3. Demonstrate your understanding about the pathophysiology in regard to the most likely diagnosis.

_____

_____

_____

_____

_____

4. Should tests/imaging studies be ordered? Which ones? Why? Think about tests/imaging beyond the primary care setting as well.

_____

_____

_____

_____

_____

5. What are the next appropriate steps in management?

_____

_____

_____

_____

6. What are the triggers, associated conditions, and treatment approaches for the diagnosis? Provide references for your responses.

_____

_____

_____

_____

7. What are the pertinent ICD-10 and CPT (E/M) codes for this visit? Provide a short rationale.

_____

_____

_____

_____

8. What is the appropriate patient education for this case?

_____

_____

_____

_____

_____

9. If not managed appropriately, what is/are the medical/legal concern(s) that may arise?

_____

_____

_____

_____

_____

10. Think about interprofessional collaboration for this case. Provide a list of specialties or other disciplines and indicate what contribution these professionals might make to managing the patient.

_____

_____

_____

_____

_____

BEDSIDE MANNER QUESTION

11. What would your communication style/approach be with this patient?

_____

_____

_____

_____

_____

ANSWER KEY _available at_
https://connect.springerpub.com/content/book/978-0-8261-8273-9

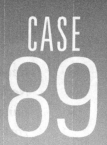

LEG PAIN, GERIATRIC MALE

CHIEF COMPLAINT
"Leg pain."

HISTORY OF PRESENT ILLNESS
A 74-year-old man, well established in this primary care clinic, presents complaining of leg pain that has been bothering him for the past few months. He states that the 4/10, crampy, calf pain in both legs occurs about 15 minutes into his twice-daily walks with his dog. The pain only goes away when he stops walking and sits for about 5 minutes. Once he starts walking again, the pain returns just a few minutes later. He also states that his legs feel weak. He reports pain relief upon elevating his legs while relaxing in his recliner but reports he sometimes cannot sleep at night as his legs start cramping when he lies down. He feels he cannot hold them still because the pain at times becomes an intense 6/10 to 7/10 until he falls asleep. He denies taking any medications for this pain but states standing in one place for an extended period, such as when fishing, also makes the pain return.

REVIEW OF SYSTEMS
The patient's ROS is positive for leg cramps and weakness, varicose veins, and arthritis in hands and feet. His ROS is negative for fainting, blackouts, seizures, weakness, paralysis, tingling, tremors, or erectile dysfunction. He denies chest pain, palpitations, dyspnea at rest or upon exertion, orthopnea, paroxysmal nocturnal dyspnea, edema, and any recent trauma to his lower extremities.

RELEVANT HISTORY
The patient has hypercholesterolemia, hypertension, and bilateral cataracts with lens implants. The patient is a retired engineer, happily married to his wife of 54 years. He is a former tobacco abuser, 2 packs per day for 30 years; he quit at age 48. He enjoys two martinis with dinner each evening and denies recreational or illicit drug use ever. His family history is significant for lung cancer, acute MI, hyperlipidemia, and hypertension.

ALLERGIES
No known drug allergies; no known food allergies.

MEDICATIONS
- Atorvastatin 40 mg PO QHS
- Amlodipine 5 mg PO QD

PHYSICAL EXAMINATION
Vitals: T 36.9°C (98.4°F), P 78, R 14, BP 146/88, HT 178 cm (70 in.), WT 82.6 kg (182 lbs), BMI 26.1.

General: Pleasant male of stated age sitting comfortably on the examination table, in no acute distress. Makes good eye contact, converses with ease, makes jokes. A&O.

Skin, Hair, and Nails: Tight, thin, shiny, atrophied skin, slightly dusky red/ruborous color, overlying dorsum of mid-feet to include all toes, extending proximally and circumferentially to bilateral ankles and knees. Bald, slightly cool to the touch bilaterally and symmetrically. No lesions or masses. Thin, short brittle nails bilateral feet.

Head: Atraumatic, normocephalic.

Neck: Trachea midline, no masses or lymphadenopathy.

Lungs: Clear to auscultation bilaterally without wheezes or rales.

Heart: RRR; no murmurs, rubs, or gallops.

Peripheral Vascular: Carotid pulses 2+ bilaterally; no thrills or bruits. Distal upper extremity pulses 2+ and symmetric bilaterally, capillary refill <2 seconds. Distal lower extremity pulses: femoral and popliteal pulses 1+ symmetric bilaterally, posterior tibial pulses 1+ symmetric bilaterally. Dorsalis pedis pulses weak bilaterally with sluggish capillary refill. Spider vein varicosities throughout BLEs. With patient lying supine, great toes blanch while lower extremities are extended and held superiorly to approximately 60°. When lower extremities are returned to the supine position, the great toes return to their original dusky red color/rubor within 6 seconds.

Musculoskeletal: FROM BUEs. LROM bilateral feet and ankles, lower extremity muscle atrophy bilaterally, most notably bilateral calves distal to feet.

Neurologic: Cranial nerves II to XII grossly intact. Negative Romberg, antalgic gait with heel-to-toe walking, walking on heels, and walking on toes.

CLINICAL DISCUSSION QUESTIONS

1. What is the differential diagnosis?

_____

_____

_____

_____

2. What is the most likely diagnosis? Why?

_____

_____

_____

_____

3. Demonstrate your understanding about the pathophysiology in regard to the most likely diagnosis.

_____

_____

_____

_____

_____

4. Should tests/imaging studies be ordered? Which ones? Why? Think about tests/imaging beyond the primary care setting as well.

_____

_____

_____

_____

_____

5. What are the next appropriate steps in management?

_____

_____

_____

_____

_____

6. What is the prevalence of the diagnosis? What is the initial diagnostic procedure for this condition? What are the treatments? Provide references for your responses.

_____

_____

_____

_____

_____

7. What are the pertinent ICD-10 and CPT (E/M) codes for this visit? Provide a short rationale.

_____

_____

_____

_____

_____

8. What is the appropriate patient education for this case?

_____

_____

_____

_____

_____

9. If not managed appropriately, what is/are the medical/legal concern(s) that may arise?

_____

_____

_____

_____

_____

10. Think about interprofessional collaboration for this case. Provide a list of specialties or other disciplines and indicate what contribution these professionals might make to managing the patient.

_____

_____

_____

_____

_____

BEDSIDE MANNER QUESTION

11. What would your communication style/approach be with this patient?

_____

_____

_____

_____

_____

ANSWER KEY available at
https://connect.springerpub.com/content/book/978-0-8261-8273-9

PAIN AND REDNESS IN BREAST, ADULT FEMALE

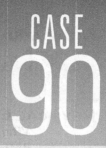

CHIEF COMPLAINT

"Pain and redness in the breast."

HISTORY OF PRESENT ILLNESS

A 50-year-old African American woman presents to her PCP with a complaint of persistent pain and redness in her left breast for the past week. She reports she first noticed the pain 4 weeks ago; however, she did not notice any skin changes at the time. One week later, she started noticing redness of the skin near and around her nipple, which made her concerned about infection. She went to a local urgent care, where she was diagnosed with cellulitis of the breast and was prescribed a 7-day course of cephalexin. She has since completed the medication and has not seen any improvement, despite taking the medication as directed and to completion. She has not noticed any worsening of the pain since it started or noticed it to be spreading.

When asked about the pain and the redness, she states that it felt and looked very similar to a bout of mastitis she experienced while breastfeeding her son years ago. She rates the pain at 6/10 and describes it as intermittent and worsened by touching the breast or with any applied pressure (like wearing her bra). She has been unable to wear her bra due to the discomfort. She denies any itching of the area and describes the pain as dull, burning, and achy without radiation beyond the breast. She denies any new exposures, including no new lotions, soaps, detergents, clothing, or foods. She denies any similar symptoms in or on her right breast. She admits to routinely performing self-breast exams at home, every month, and denies any masses or lumps in the breasts or axilla.

REVIEW OF SYSTEMS

The patient's ROS is positive for skin "rash" to left breast, increased warmth, and pain to affected area, pain in the left shoulder, with limited range of motion due to "tightness." Her ROS is negative for fever, chills, weight loss, breast lumps, vomiting, headache, weakness, abdominal pain, cough, SOB, chest wall pain, acid reflux, easy bruising or bleeding, and bone or joint pain.

RELEVANT HISTORY

The patient's medical history is unremarkable, without any diagnosed adult illnesses. She is up to date on all vaccinations. She has never had surgery but had two overnight hospitalizations for the birth of her sons. Her last physical exam was 7 months ago, with routine labs performed for anemia and cholesterol, which were normal. She was referred for mammogram and colonoscopy at that time but has not yet scheduled these tests. She is in menopause. She has been married to her female partner for the past 18 years and is happy in her relationship. She and her partner are sexually active in a monogamous relationship, and she had no previous sexual partners prior to this relationship. She was tested for all STIs, including HIV, about 10 years ago, all of which were negative.

ALLERGIES

No known drug, food, or environmental allergies.

MEDICATIONS

- Famotidine 20 mg QD PRN for heartburn
- Vitamin B12 QD

PHYSICAL EXAMINATION

Vitals: T 37.5°C (99.5°F), P 90, R 14, BP 118/78, HT 165 cm (64 in.), WT 60.7 kg (134 lbs), BMI 23.0.

General: Nervous-appearing female, mildly uncomfortable but nontoxic appearing.

Psychiatric: Appears nervous and worried but calm and cooperative.

Skin, Hair, and Nails: General skin exam reveals dark brown color (Fitzpatrick V), unremarkable except for a small keloid scar on her right thigh and a few scattered skin tags on her superior aspect of upper back/superior shoulder areas. Large patch-like area of violaceous/pink skin on dark brown skin tone, dimpled and rough in texture on left breast 1 cm from areola, circumferential to areola and extending to mid-breast with tenderness to palpation and increased warmth and pitting. No induration or drainage from lesion or nipple. Right breast without skin changes. No abnormal findings with hair or nails.

ENT/Mouth: Nares patent, oropharynx clear.

Neck: No cervical/supraclavicular/occipital lymphadenopathy. No nodules or lumps palpable.

Breasts: Pendulous breasts bilateral, with asymmetry of left breast resting more superficial to right breast. Skin as noted previously. No palpable lumps or masses in either breast. Nipples without deformity or drainage. Left breast tender to palpation over affected violaceous/pink area with large area of induration near areola. No palpable lymphadenopathy in bilateral axilla.

Lungs: Clear to auscultation bilaterally without wheezes/rhonchi/crackles.

Heart: RRR without murmur.

Abdomen: Soft, non-tender, not distended, active bowel sounds throughout.

Musculoskeletal: Limited flexion and abduction of left shoulder due to tightness referred from left breast with active ROM. FROM passively on left shoulder.

Neurologic: A&O×3, cranial nerves II to XII intact.

CLINICAL DISCUSSION QUESTIONS

1. What is the differential diagnosis?

_____

_____

_____

_____

_____

2. What is the most likely diagnosis? Why?

_____

_____

_____

_____

_____

3. Demonstrate your understanding about the pathophysiology in regard to the most likely diagnosis.

_____

_____

_____

_____

4. Should tests/imaging studies be ordered? Which ones? Why? Think about tests/imaging beyond the primary care setting as well.

_____

_____

_____

_____

5. What are the next appropriate steps in management?

_____

_____

_____

_____

6. What are the diagnostic challenges, diagnostic studies, and disparities in race and socioeconomic factors of the diagnosis? Provide references for your response.

_____

_____

_____

_____

7. What are the pertinent ICD-10 and CPT (E/M) codes for this visit? Provide a short rationale.

_____

_____

_____

_____

8. What are the appropriate patient education topics for this case?

_____

_____

_____

_____

9. If not managed appropriately, what is/are the medical/legal concern(s) that may arise?

_____

_____

_____

_____

10. Think about interprofessional collaboration for this case. Provide a list of specialties or other disciplines and indicate what contribution these professionals might make to managing the patient.

_____

_____

_____

_____

BEDSIDE MANNER QUESTIONS

11. What would your communication style/approach be with this patient?

_____

_____

_____

12. If the patient shows distress at what you communicate, how would you provide support?

_____

_____

_____

_____

ANSWER KEY _available at_
https://connect.springerpub.com/content/book/978-0-8261-8273-9

STOMACH PAIN AND BLOATING, ADOLESCENT FEMALE

CHIEF COMPLAINT

"Stomach pain with bloating."

HISTORY OF PRESENT ILLNESS

A 17-year-old young woman accompanied by her mother presents to her regular PCP with concerns of abdominal pain, bloating, and diarrhea over the past 6 months. The patient noticed worsening abdominal pain and diarrhea several days ago. She continues to have abdominal bloating and cramping with foul-smelling, watery diarrhea and flatus 7 days afterward. She tried bismuth subsalicylate and loperamide for diarrhea with little relief. She has missed multiple school days because of her abdominal pain and diarrhea. The patient has been on a lactose-free diet for 2 months with no improvement of her symptoms. She also stopped soft drinks and fast food. According to her mother, she has been more tired and moody for several months. Her last menstrual cycle was a week ago. She denies sexual activity for over 6 months and has had no recent travel.

REVIEW OF SYSTEMS

The patient's ROS is positive for unintentional weight loss of 10 lbs, chronic fatigue, arthralgias, itchy rash on anterior lower legs, rhinorrhea, canker sores, abdominal pain, bloating, vomiting, occasional dyspepsia, persistent diarrhea, and moodiness. Her ROS is negative for fever, chills, nausea, changes in appetite, dysuria, pelvic pain, abnormal vaginal discharge or bleeding, rectal bleeding, melena, hematochezia, hematuria, sexual activity, or STIs. She denies anxiety or depression.

RELEVANT HISTORY

The patient had recurrent tonsillitis when she was younger, which resolved with tonsillectomy at age 8, acute appendicitis at age 12, and a fracture of left foot 4 months ago. Her mother has IBS and type 1 diabetes, and her father and two brothers have no health conditions. She has a maternal aunt with celiac sprue and a maternal grandmother diagnosed with celiac sprue, type 1 diabetes, and thyroid disease.

ALLERGIES

No known drug allergies; no known food allergies.

MEDICATIONS

None.

PHYSICAL EXAMINATION

Vitals: T 37°C (98.6°F), P 74, R 14, BP 100/68, HT 160.02 cm (63 in.), WT 49.90 kg (110 lbs), BMI 19.5.

General: Patient appears in no acute distress, well developed, pale in appearance.

Psychiatric: Normal mood and affect.

Skin, Hair, and Nails: Papulovesicular rash on extensor surface with mild excoriations located on bilateral lower legs. Normal skin turgor. No abnormal findings with hair or nails.

Eyes: Conjunctivae are pale.

ENT/Mouth: TM appear pearly gray with normal landmarks; nose with boggy turbinates and clear rhinorrhea; oral mucosa is moist; no ulcerations, no oropharyngeal erythema; tonsils are absent; several dental caries in upper and lower molars.

Lungs: Clear to auscultation bilaterally.

Heart: RRR, with no murmurs, gallops, or rubs.

Abdomen: Soft, mildly distended with no masses, guarding, or rigidity. No hepatosplenomegaly. Negative Murphy sign, McBurney point, and psoas and obturator tests.

Musculoskeletal: No joint swelling or tenderness; ROM of all joints are normal.

Genital/Rectal: No perianal skin tags, fistulas, or abscess. No masses or retained stool on digital rectal exam. Negative occult fecal blood testing.

CLINICAL DISCUSSION QUESTIONS

1. What is the differential diagnosis?

_____

_____

_____

_____

2. What is the most likely diagnosis? Why?

_____

_____

_____

_____

_____

3. Demonstrate your understanding about the pathophysiology in regard to the most likely diagnosis.

_____

_____

_____

_____

_____

4. Should tests/imaging studies be ordered? Which ones? Why? Think about tests/imaging beyond the primary care setting as well.

_____

_____

_____

_____

_____

5. What are the next appropriate steps in management?

_____

_____

_____

_____

_____

6. Review reliable, recent references and demonstrate an understanding of the diagnostic approach, treatment, and follow-up recommendations for this diagnosis. Include the name of the source(s).

_____

_____

_____

_____

_____

7. What are the pertinent ICD-10 and CPT (E/M) codes for this visit? Provide a short rationale.

_____

_____

_____

_____

_____

8. What are appropriate patient/family education topics for this case?

_____

_____

_____

_____

_____

9. If not managed appropriately, what is/are the medical/legal concern(s) that may arise?

_____

_____

_____

_____

_____

10. Think about interprofessional collaboration for this case. Provide a list of specialties or other disciplines and indicate what contribution these professionals might make to managing the patient.

_____

_____

_____

_____

_____

BEDSIDE MANNER QUESTION
11. What would your communication style/approach be with this patient and parent?

_____

_____

_____

_____

_____

ANSWER KEY _available at_
https://connect.springerpub.com/content/book/978-0-8261-8273-9

REDNESS ON LOWER RIGHT LEG, ADULT MALE

CHIEF COMPLAINT

"Redness on lower leg."

HISTORY OF PRESENT ILLNESS

A 35-year-old man presents to the clinic for the first time with a 3-day complaint of worsening pain and redness noted to the right lower extremity. He is a landscaper who states "something bit me" while working. He noticed the bushes were full of spider webs and insects. He describes a slight pain to his right leg that developed 3 days later, with a reddened area and a small pin poke to the center. He reports pain as 5/10, increased with movement of his right leg, with no numbness or tingling. He wears long protective clothing, wears high boots when working, and has had no previous problems. He has tried OTC cream with no relief of symptoms; medication name unknown.

REVIEW OF SYSTEMS

The patient's ROS is positive for pain, tenderness, rash, and redness to lower right leg. The ROS is negative for recent travel (including flights or long car rides), itchiness, fever, chills, nausea, vomiting, malaise, confusion, headache, SOB, or chest pain.

RELEVANT HISTORY

The patient's relevant history includes chronic back pain and hypertension. He currently takes blood pressure medication. The patient lives alone and is a social smoker on the weekends (cigars and cigarettes). He drinks 1 to 2 beers during the week and a 12-pack on the weekends. His family history includes diabetes, hypertension, and chronic kidney disease on the paternal side and breast cancer and hypertension on the maternal side. He has two siblings, who are alive and healthy.

ALLERGIES

No known drug allergies; no known food allergies.

MEDICATIONS

Lisinopril 10 mg PO QD.

PHYSICAL EXAMINATION

Vitals: T 99.7°C (37.7°F), P 74, R 16, BP 148/86, WT 114.75 kg (253 lbs), HT 172.7 cm (58 in.), BMI 38.5.

General: A&O; calm, cooperative, well groomed, well nourished.

Skin, Hair, and Nails: Skin intact, warm to touch; hair is equally dispersed to arms and lower extremities. Right lower extremity with tenderness to moderate palpation, mild edema on the distal/posterior lower extremity, and erythema; no difference between the right and left calf measurements; well-demarcated small tiny puncture bite to distal/posterior right lower extremity; circular rash 10 cm × 6.5 cm. No drainage. Skin is tight and shiny to epidermis of skin. No vesicles, not pruritic. Capillary refill < 2 seconds bilaterally. No abnormal findings with hair or nails.

Heart: RRR, no murmur, pedal pulses palpable.

Lungs: Clear to auscultation bilaterally.

Musculoskeletal: FROM of right ankle/foot, red, warm, and tender to touch. Normal ROM to left foot.

Neurologic: Achilles reflexes 2+ bilaterally, limited dorsiflexion of right foot, pain with dorsiflexion, no paresthesia, limping gait.

CLINICAL DISCUSSION QUESTIONS

1. What is the differential diagnosis?

_____

_____

_____

_____

_____

2. What is the most likely diagnosis? Why?

_____

_____

_____

_____

_____

3. Demonstrate your understanding about the pathophysiology in regard to the most likely diagnosis.

_____

_____

_____

_____

_____

4. Should tests/imaging studies be ordered? Which ones? Why? Think about tests/imaging beyond the primary care setting as well.

_____

_____

_____

_____

_____

5. What are the next appropriate steps in management?

_____

_____

_____

_____

6. What are the diagnosis and treatment approaches for this condition? Discuss common misdiagnoses for this condition. Provide references for your responses.

_____

_____

_____

_____

_____

7. What are the pertinent ICD-10 and CPT (E/M) codes for this visit? Provide a short rationale.

_____

_____

_____

_____

_____

8. What is the appropriate patient education for this case?

_____

_____

_____

_____

_____

9. If not managed appropriately, what is/are the medical/legal concern(s) that may arise?

_____

_____

_____

_____

_____

10. Think about interprofessional collaboration for this case. Provide a list of specialties or other disciplines and indicate what contribution these professionals might make to managing the patient.

_____

_____

_____

_____

_____

BEDSIDE MANNER QUESTION
11. What would your communication style/approach be with this patient?

_____

_____

_____

_____

 ANSWER KEY *available at*
https://connect.springerpub.com/content/book/978-0-8261-8273-9

BLOOD IN STOOL, ADULT FEMALE

CHIEF COMPLAINT
"Blood in stool."

HISTORY OF PRESENT ILLNESS

A 52-year-old woman with obesity and hypothyroidism presents to an urgent care clinic affiliated with her PCP's practice for rectal bleeding for the past 4 months. Initially, it happened about once a week during a bowel movement but was currently occurring daily with all bowel movements. She describes the blood as approximately 1 teaspoon, dark red, and mixed in the stool. She denies any associated rectal or abdominal pain, and her bowel movements are regular every day without change, although they do seem thinner, which she attributes to starting a low-carbohydrate diet 4 months ago. She relays a history of internal hemorrhoids after the birth of her daughter 20 years ago, with rare bleeding throughout the years that always improves within a day of applying over-the-counter hemorrhoid cream. Despite using this cream daily now, there has been no improvement in current symptoms. Though she was referred for colonoscopy screening at age 50, she never scheduled it because she was "afraid of the prep" and did not want to miss a whole day of work. She states she called her regular PCP 3 months ago about her bleeding. "He told to me that my insurance allows me to see the gastroenterologist without a referral, so I should go there and get a colonoscopy done." The procedure is scheduled in 3 weeks, the earliest available for the "routine screening" referral sent. The patient asked whether "the take-home test" or a "virtual colonoscopy" could be ordered today for quicker results.

REVIEW OF SYSTEMS

The patient endorses fatigue and weight loss of 12 lbs in 4 months, which she attributes to dieting, and occasional night sweats, which she attributes to menopause. She denies fever or chills. She endorses increasing SOB when walking upstairs or hills for the past month but denies any chest pain, palpitations, or syncope; endorses dizziness when standing up quickly but denies headache, weakness, or paresthesia; denies cough, wheezing, or hemoptysis; denies anorexia, heartburn, nausea/vomiting, diarrhea, or melena; denies any dysuria, hematuria, vaginal bleeding or discharge, or pelvic pain; denies any increased bruising or swollen lymph nodes; denies any skin rashes, lesions, or itching; and denies insomnia, anxiety, or depression.

RELEVANT HISTORY

The patient has struggled with obesity since her pregnancy at age 32, after which she was diagnosed with hypothyroidism. She has taken levothyroxine 112 mcg daily for 20 years but takes no other medications or supplements. She has no prior history of heart, lung, GI, or bleeding disorders, and she has no prior surgeries or hospitalizations.

Her parents are alive and healthy in their late 70s; she believes her maternal grandmother died in her 60s of "some kind of stomach cancer." There is no family history of heart disease, diabetes, or bleeding disorder.

She is married and sexually active. She does not smoke or use any recreational drugs. She drinks 2 glasses of wine every night with dinner.

ALLERGIES

None.

MEDICATIONS

Levothyroxine 112 mcg QD.

PHYSICAL EXAMINATION

Vitals: T 37.2°C (99.0°F), P 98, R 18, BP 110/62, SPo$_2$ 97%, HT 157.5 cm (62 in.), WT 91.2 kg (201 lbs), BMI 36.0.

General: Well-developed, obese Caucasian female; A&O; all vital signs stable; in no acute distress.

Psychiatric: Broad affect euthymic mood, fluent speech, average insight.

Skin, Hair, and Nails: Warm and dry, pallor of skin noted, nail beds, and conjunctivae. No jaundice or rashes present. No abnormal findings with hair or nails.

Lungs: Clear to auscultation bilaterally with no adventitious sounds. Good effort with no accessory muscle use.

Heart: RRR with no murmurs, gallops, or rubs.

Abdomen: Protuberant noted with central obesity. Normal active bowel sounds in all quadrants with no bruits noted. Soft, non-tender, non-distended; no masses, organomegaly, or hernia present.

Genital/Rectal: Genital exam deferred; rectal exam shows normal sphincter tone, no fissures noted, visible small non-tender non-thrombosed external hemorrhoid visible at 6 o' clock, and a small non-tender internal hemorrhoid at 9 o' clock. Brown hard stool and gross blood noted in vault, which is guaiac-fecal occult blood test positive.

Extremities: No edema, clubbing, or cyanosis. Radial and dorsalis pedis pulses 2+ bilaterally.

Neurologic: Gait steady; no tremors, no focal deficits.

CLINICAL DISCUSSION QUESTIONS

1. What is the differential diagnosis?

_____

_____

_____

_____

2. What is the most likely diagnosis? Why?

_____

_____

_____

_____

3. Demonstrate your understanding about the pathophysiology in regard to the most likely diagnosis.

_____

_____

_____

_____

4. Should tests/imaging studies be ordered? Which ones? Why? Think about tests/imaging beyond the primary care setting as well.

_____

_____

_____

_____

5. What are the next appropriate steps in management?

_____

_____

_____

_____

6. What are the incidence and screening recommendations for this diagnosis? Provide references for your response.

_____

_____

_____

_____

7. What are the pertinent ICD-10 and CPT (E/M) codes for this visit? Provide a short rationale.

_____

_____

_____

_____

8. What is the appropriate patient education for this case?

_____

_____

_____

_____

9. If not managed appropriately, what is/are the medical/legal concern(s) that may arise?

_____

_____

_____

_____

10. Think about interprofessional collaboration for this case. Provide a list of specialties or other disciplines and indicate what contribution these professionals might make to managing the patient.

_____

_____

_____

_____

BEDSIDE MANNER QUESTION
11. What would your communication style/approach be with this patient?

_____

_____

_____

_____

ANSWER KEY _available at_
https://connect.springerpub.com/content/book/978-0-8261-8273-9

ERECTION DIFFICULTIES, ADULT MALE

CHIEF COMPLAINT

"Erection difficulties."

HISTORY OF PRESENT ILLNESS

A 23-year-old cisgender man presents to his PCP with a 7-day history of inability to have an erection. He states this has never happened before. The patient had sex with a partner the night before his symptoms started and was fine. He denies any trauma to his penis or any pain during sexual activity. He has talked to his friends about it and was told it was probably stress related. He reports infrequent marijuana use and two nights weekly of drinking, 6 drinks a night. He has been smoking 2 to 3 cigarettes per day for the last 3 years. He does not believe the erection difficulties occurred because of alcohol or marijuana use. The patient reports he gets enough sleep. He reports no changes in urinary function or flow. He denies any rectal pain or pressure. He states he still has morning erections but not as hard as usual. He denies changes in his interest in or response to sexual arousal. He does report significant life stress from school and exams and has a history of depression. He denies any previous STI testing or diagnosis but would like to be tested and reports a total of three to four male partners in his lifetime. The patient engages in receptive anal intercourse (condoms sometimes) and oral sex with no condoms. His last sexual contact was 8 days ago, when he had receptive anal intercourse with no condom.

REVIEW OF SYSTEMS

The patient's ROS is positive for erectile dysfunction and stress. His ROS is negative for lack of appetite, lack of energy, lack of concentration, anxiety, fever, chills, dysuria, urinary urgency, hematuria, penile discharge, rash, SOB, or chest pain.

RELEVANT HISTORY

The patient has a history of depression and attention deficit disorder. He is a graduate student in architecture. No significant family medical history.

ALLERGIES

No known drug allergies; no known food allergies.

MEDICATIONS

None.

PHYSICAL EXAMINATION

Vitals: T 36.4°C (97.6°F), P 69, R 16, BP 112/70, HT 170 cm (67 in.), WT 60.3 kg (133 lbs), BMI 20.8.

General: Vital signs stable, no acute distress.

Psychiatric: Engaged but distant (not comfortable talking about this today). Appears anxious.

Genital/Rectal: Rectal exam deferred. Genitourinary exam revealed healthy-appearing circumcised penis. No edema, discharge, or erythema. There were also no ulcers or lesions. Chaperone for this exam was offered and declined by patient.

CLINICAL DISCUSSION QUESTIONS

1. What is the differential diagnosis?

_____

_____

_____

_____

_____

2. What is the most likely diagnosis? Why?

_____

_____

_____

_____

_____

3. Demonstrate your understanding regarding the pathophysiology of the most likely diagnosis.

_____

_____

_____

_____

_____

4. Should tests/imaging studies be ordered? Which ones? Why? Think about tests/imaging beyond the primary care setting as well.

_____

_____

_____

_____

_____

5. What are the next appropriate steps in management?

_____

_____

_____

_____

_____

6. What are the prevalence and contributing factors of this diagnosis in young adult males? What is a first-line recommendation to help treat this condition without medication? Provide references for your answers.

_____

_____

_____

_____

_____

_____

7. What are the pertinent ICD-10 and CPT (E/M) codes for this visit? Provide a short rationale.

_____

_____

_____

_____

_____

8. What is the appropriate patient education for this case?

_____

_____

_____

_____

9. If not managed appropriately, what is/are the medical/legal concern(s) that may arise?

_____

_____

_____

_____

_____

10. Think about interprofessional collaboration for this case. Provide a list of specialties or other disciplines and indicate what contribution these professionals might make to managing the patient.

_____

_____

_____

_____

_____

BEDSIDE MANNER QUESTION

11. What would your communication style/approach be with this patient?

_____

_____

_____

_____

_____

ANSWER KEY *available at*
https://connect.springerpub.com/content/book/978-0-8261-8273-9

REFUSAL TO EAT OR DRINK, PEDIATRIC MALE

CHIEF COMPLAINT
"Refusal to eat or drink."

HISTORY OF PRESENT ILLNESS
A mother brings her 5-year-old son to his PCP for evaluation of a 2-day refusal to eat and drink. The mother reports the child has been extremely fussy; he has not been sleeping well, wakes up crying, and is hard to console. The mother states the child was hot to touch but she was unable to measure his temperature, because she does not have a thermometer. She has been giving him children's acetaminophen and diphenhydramine to help with fussiness and sleep. The mother denies vomiting or diarrhea by the child. She adds he was well and active 2 days ago. The mother denies sick contact with his other sibling but did note that there are other children at day care with similar symptoms.

REVIEW OF SYSTEMS
The patient's ROS is positive for fever, excessive irritability, refusal to eat or drink, and fatigue. His ROS is negative for vomiting, diarrhea, abdominal pain, headache, difficulty talking, runny nose, or persistent cough.

RELEVANT HISTORY
The child's medical history is significant for a full-term birth at 39 weeks without pregnancy complications. His immunizations are up to date. He has no history of hospitalizations and no chronic medical conditions. He has met all developmental milestones and growth trajectories without concern. He lives with his parents, attends pre-K day care full-time, and eats a balanced diet. His mother and father are healthy. They have no chronic medical conditions.

ALLERGIES
No known drug, food, or environmental allergies.

MEDICATIONS
None.

PHYSICAL EXAMINATION
Vitals: T 38.4°C (101.2°F), P 118, R 20, BP 110/80, HT 109.2 (43 in.), WT 19.1 kg (42 lbs), BMI 16.

General: Alert, fussy and irritable, seems fatigued.

Skin, Hair, and Nails: No abnormal findings. No rash.

Head: Normocephalic and atraumatic.

ENT/Mouth: Oropharyngeal and tonsillar area with moderate beefy red erythema with white exudates; no stridor noted; no uvular deviation noted; patient is tolerating oral secretions; no tripod position noted. Surface of the oral mucosa and tongue without abnormal findings.

Neck: Neck is soft, supple, with adequate ROM; no nuchal rigidity noted; tender adenopathy in anterior and posterior cervical chain present.

Lungs: Clear to auscultation bilaterally with equal and symmetrical respiratory excursion.

Heart: RRR; no murmur or gallops noted.

Abdomen: Soft, not distended, appears non-tender.

Neurologic: Cranial nerves II to XII are grossly intact; no problem with gait or balance noted.

CLINICAL DISCUSSION QUESTIONS

1. What is the differential diagnosis?

_____

_____

_____

_____

_____

2. What is the most likely diagnosis? Why?

_____

_____

_____

_____

_____

3. Demonstrate your understanding about the pathophysiology in regard to the most likely diagnosis.

_____

_____

_____

_____

_____

4. Should tests/imaging studies be ordered? Which ones? Why? Think about tests/imaging beyond the primary care setting as well.

_____

_____

_____

_____

_____

5. What are the next appropriate steps in management?

6. What is the most common cause of and treatment for this diagnosis in children, and what are the risks associated with a missed diagnosis? Provide references for your response.

7. What are the pertinent ICD-10 and CPT (E/M) codes for this visit? Provide a short rationale.

8. What are the appropriate parent education topics for this case?

9. If not managed appropriately, what is/are the medical/legal concern(s) that may arise?

10. Think about interprofessional collaboration for this case. Provide a list of specialties or other disciplines and indicate what contribution these professionals might make to managing the patient.

_____

_____

_____

_____

_____

BEDSIDE MANNER QUESTION
11. What would your communication style/approach be with this parent?

_____

_____

_____

_____

_____

ANSWER KEY *available at*
https://connect.springerpub.com/content/book/978-0-8261-8273-9

UNEXPLAINED WEIGHT GAIN, ADULT FEMALE

CHIEF COMPLAINT

"Unexplained weight gain."

HISTORY OF PRESENT ILLNESS

A 34-year-old Caucasian woman presents to her PCP with a 1-year history of weight gain despite efforts to eat healthy and increase physical activity. She is married and a mother of three children, 13-year-old twin boys and a 6-year-old girl. She states she did not pay attention to the gradual weight gain until about 4 months ago, when she began making efforts to lose weight to include walking and eating less fast food.

REVIEW OF SYSTEMS

The patient's ROS is positive for a 25-lb weight gain over the past year. Her last menstrual period was 2 weeks ago. Her ROS is negative for fatigue, dry skin, acne, fever, thinning hair, hypertension, swelling, weakness, reduced exercise tolerance, abdominal pain or distension, constipation, excessive hair growth, nipple discharge, anxiety, depression, substance abuse concerns, cold intolerance, difficulty sleeping, snoring, joint pain, polydipsia, or polyuria.

RELEVANT HISTORY

The patient's relevant history includes vitamin D deficiency. She smokes half a pack of cigarettes per day. The patient admits she is less active than she used to be and consumes a diet high in carbohydrates. She denies alcohol or illicit drug use. She lives with her husband and describes it as stressful. Her family history is positive for type 2 diabetes mellitus, hypertension, hyperlipidemia, and early heart disease.

ALLERGIES

No known drug allergies; no known food allergies.

MEDICATIONS

- OTC multivitamin daily.
- Vitamin D 50,000 IU weekly.

PHYSICAL EXAMINATION

Vitals: T 36.7°C (98.1°F), P 70, R 18, BP 116/77, HT 170 cm (67 in.), WT 93 kg (205 lbs), BMI 32.1.

General: Obese and well groomed in no acute distress.

Psychiatric: Normal mood and affect.

Skin, Hair, and Nails: Skin warm and dry with no excessive facial hair or rash. No abnormal findings with nails.

Neck: Thyroid is normal size; consistency and is non-tender.

Lungs: Clear to auscultation bilaterally.

Heart: RRR, radial pulse 2+ bilaterally.

Lymphatic: Nonpalpable cervical nodes

Abdomen: Rounded, non-distended, soft, non-tender, normal bowel sounds.

Musculoskeletal: No extremity edema. FROM both upper and lower extremities, bilateral.

Neurologic: A&O×3 without tics or tremors.

CLINICAL DISCUSSION QUESTIONS

1. What is the differential diagnosis?

_____

_____

_____

_____

_____

2. What is the most likely diagnosis? Why?

_____

_____

_____

_____

3. Demonstrate your understanding about the pathophysiology in regard to the most likely diagnosis.

_____

_____

_____

_____

4. Should tests/imaging studies be ordered? Which ones? Why? Think about tests/imaging beyond the primary care setting as well.

_____

_____

_____

_____

5. What are the next appropriate steps in management?

_____

_____

_____

_____

_____

6. What are the diagnostic criteria and risk factors for this diagnosis? Provide references for your response.

_____

_____

_____

_____

_____

7. What are the pertinent ICD-10 and CPT (E/M) codes for this visit? Provide a short rationale.

_____

_____

_____

_____

_____

8. What is the appropriate patient education for this case?

_____

_____

_____

_____

9. If not managed appropriately, what is/are the medical/legal concern(s) that may arise?

_____

_____

_____

_____

10. Think about interprofessional collaboration for this case. Provide a list of specialties or other disciplines and indicate what contribution these professionals might make to managing the patient.

_____

_____

_____

_____

_____

BEDSIDE MANNER QUESTIONS

11. What would your communication style/approach be with this patient?

_____

_____

_____

_____

_____

12. If the patient shows distress at what you communicate, how would you provide support?

_____

_____

_____

_____

_____

ANSWER KEY _available at_
https://connect.springerpub.com/content/book/978-0-8261-8273-9

WORSENING, SHARP ABDOMINAL PAIN, ADULT FEMALE

CHIEF COMPLAINT

"Worsening, sharp abdominal pain."

HISTORY OF PRESENT ILLNESS

A 22-year-old woman presents as a new patient to the primary care clinic, complaining of abdominal pain for the past week and a half. The pain became worse while having sexual intercourse with her boyfriend today. She states she had intercourse around 2.5 hours prior to arrival. She describes the pain as sharp in nature, located in the suprapubic region, rated 8/10, and constant; but it does not radiate, although she also has lower back pain. Her last menstrual period was almost 3 weeks ago. Her cycles are noted to be regular and last approximately 3 days. She states she has never experienced this type of pain before. The pain is exacerbated by movement and sexual intercourse, and she denies any relieving factors. She states she is currently in a monogamous relationship with her boyfriend of 2 years, and they do not use any form of contraception.

REVIEW OF SYSTEMS

The patient's ROS is positive for suprapubic pain, low back pain, dyspareunia, nausea, fever, chills, frequency, and yellow-white vaginal discharge. The ROS is negative for vomiting, diarrhea, urgency, dysuria, anorexia, chest pain, SOB, headaches, dizziness, and abnormal vaginal bleeding.

RELEVANT HISTORY

The patient is a full-time graduate student who lives alone. She has never been pregnant, denies tobacco use, drinks a glass of wine socially approximately two to three times a month, and denies recreational drug use. She has a history of trichomonas diagnosed and treated at age 18.

ALLERGIES

No known drug allergies; no known food allergies.

MEDICATIONS

OTC daily multivitamin.

PHYSICAL EXAMINATION

Vitals: T 37.7°C (99.9°F), P 67, R 18, BP 127/86, SpO$_2$ 98%, HT 167.64 cm (66 in.), WT 90.72 kg (200 lbs), BMI 32.27.

General: Ill-appearing obese female lying in the right lateral decubitus position, in moderate distress secondary to pain.

Skin, Hair, and Nails: No visible rash; no abnormal findings on hair or nails.

Psychiatric: Cooperative, slightly anxious, likely secondary to pain.

Chest: Normal anteroposterior diameter, symmetric chest wall expansion, no chest wall tenderness to palpation.

Lungs: Breath sounds clear to auscultation bilaterally, without wheezing, rales, or rhonchi.

Heart: RRR, S1, S2, no murmurs, rubs, or gallops.

Abdomen: Non-distended, normal active bowel sounds, soft, tenderness noted in the right lower quadrant, no guarding, no rebound, no masses appreciated; psoas, rovsing, and obturator signs all negative.

Genital/Rectal: Normal external genitalia without rash, ulcerations, nodularities, or abnormal lesions. Speculum exam notes moist, pink, vaginal walls with mild erythema, frothy, thin, yellow-white discharge pooled in the posterior fornix noted; no lesions or ulcerations. Cervix is erythematous, with noted discharge. Cervical motion tenderness noted. Bimanual exam notes positive bilateral adnexal tenderness to palpation, with no palpable masses appreciated. Rectal exam notes no lesions or ulcerations, normal sphincter tone, not tender to palpation. No palpable inguinal lymphadenopathy. Genital/rectal exam was performed with a chaperone (MA) present in the room.

Musculoskeletal: Negative bilateral costovertebral angle tenderness.

Neurologic: A&O×3. Cranial nerves II to XII grossly intact.

CLINICAL DISCUSSION QUESTIONS

1. What is the differential diagnosis?

_____

_____

_____

_____

2. What is the most likely diagnosis? Why?

_____

_____

_____

_____

3. Demonstrate your understanding about the pathophysiology in regard to the most likely diagnosis.

_____

_____

_____

_____

4. Should tests/imaging studies be ordered? Which ones? Why? Think about tests/imaging beyond the primary care setting as well.

_____

_____

_____

_____

5. What are the next appropriate steps in management?

_____

_____

_____

_____

6. What are the adverse outcomes and treatment recommendations for this diagnosis and its relationship to trichomonas? List the name of your references.

_____

_____

_____

_____

7. What are the pertinent ICD-10 and CPT (E/M) codes for this visit? Provide a short rationale.

_____

_____

_____

_____

8. What are the appropriate patient education topics for this case?

_____

_____

_____

_____

9. If not managed appropriately, what is/are the medical/legal concern(s) that may arise?

_____

_____

_____

_____

_____

10. Think about interprofessional collaboration for this case. Provide a list of specialties or other disciplines and indicate what contribution these professionals might make to managing the patient.

_____

_____

_____

_____

_____

BEDSIDE MANNER QUESTION

11. What would your communication style/approach be with this patient?

_____

_____

_____

_____

_____

 ANSWER KEY _available at_
https://connect.springerpub.com/content/book/978-0-8261-8273-9

LUMP IN BREAST, ADULT MALE

CHIEF COMPLAINT

"Lump in breast."

HISTORY OF PRESENT ILLNESS

A 42-year-old, generally healthy man presents for evaluation of a mass on his right chest wall/breast. He states he has a "hard nodule" below his right nipple that he noticed 2 days ago; it is not painful and has not changed. He denies trauma or injury to the area. He reports no galactorrhea or bleeding from the nipple or skin and no skin changes on the chest. He denies any masses anywhere else on his body. He denies any systemic symptoms such as weight changes, fevers, or night sweats. He has never had anything like this before; nothing makes it better or worse, and he has not tried any medication or treatment at this time.

REVIEW OF SYSTEMS

A ROS is positive for breast mass and a history of moderate erectile dysfunction after a vascular injury to his penis several years ago, and he states his erectile dysfunction may have worsened recently. The ROS is negative for skin lesions; chills or sweats; fatigue, malaise, or weakness; polyuria; polydipsia; polyphagia; heat or cold intolerance; change in voice, hair, or skin; excessive sweating or weight change; easy bruising or bleeding; abdominal pain; early satiety; changes in appetite or bowel habits; dysuria; obstructive voiding symptoms; testicular pain; swelling or testicular mass; or urethral discharge.

RELEVANT HISTORY

The patient's medical history is significant for carcinoma of the thyroid, with a total thyroidectomy and radiation treatment (age 16); traumatic vascular injury to penis/urethra with subsequent scarring, resulting in erectile dysfunction (age 22); and vasectomy without complications (age 40). His social history includes alcohol use (4 drinks/week), no tobacco use, and regular exercise. He is a firefighter, married with one child (age 7). His family history is significant for bladder cancer in father (age 56), breast cancer in paternal grandmother (age 59), ovarian cancer in a paternal aunt (age 43), lung cancer in maternal grandmother (age 75), and bone cancer in his maternal grandfather (age 55).

ALLERGIES

No known drug allergies; no known food allergies.

MEDICATIONS

- Levothyroxine 175 mcg QD.
- Sildenafil 25 mg PRN.

PHYSICAL EXAMINATION

Vitals: T 37°C (98.6°F), P 54, R 16, BP 140/83; HT 178 cm (70 in.), WT 70 kg (155 lbs), BMI 22.

General: Well-developed, well-nourished male in no apparent distress; appears fit; appears stated age.

Neck: Faint thyroidectomy scar across the anterior neck; no palpable thyroid tissue or neck mass noted; no cervical adenopathy or tenderness bilaterally.

Lungs: Clear to auscultation bilaterally without wheezes, rales, or rhonchi.

Breast: Right-sided retro-areolar non-tender breast mass palpated, firm, smooth, and mobile, approximately 3 cm in diameter without skin changes or retraction of the nipple; no erythema or warmth; no galactorrhea; left breast with no abnormal findings; no axillary or supraclavicular adenopathy bilaterally.

Heart: RRR without murmur, rubs, or gallops.

Abdomen: Soft, flat, non-tender; positive bowel sounds; no masses, no hepatosplenomegaly.

Genital/Rectal: Circumcised penis with midline urethra; no plaques, no urethral discharge; scrotum without swelling or tenderness; testes palpated without masses or tenderness bilaterally. Rectal exam deferred.

CLINICAL DISCUSSION QUESTIONS

1. What is the differential diagnosis?

_____

_____

_____

_____

2. What is the most likely diagnosis? Why?

_____

_____

_____

_____

3. Demonstrate your understanding about the pathophysiology in regard to the most likely diagnosis.

_____

_____

_____

_____

4. Should tests/imaging studies be ordered? Which ones? Why? Think about tests/imaging beyond the primary care setting as well.

_____

_____

_____

_____

5. What are the next appropriate steps in management?

_____

_____

_____

_____

6. What are the causes of this diagnosis and the most helpful diagnostic imaging studies for the initial workup? Why thorough follow-up is vital for this diagnosis? Provide references for your response.

_____

_____

_____

_____

7. What are the pertinent ICD-10 and CPT (E/M) codes for this visit? Provide a short rationale.

_____

_____

_____

_____

8. What is the appropriate patient education topic for this case?

_____

_____

_____

_____

9. If not managed appropriately, what is/are the medical/legal concern(s) that may arise?

_____

_____

_____

_____

10. Think about interprofessional collaboration for this case. Provide a list of specialties or other disciplines and indicate what contribution these professionals might make to managing the patient.

_____

_____

_____

_____

BEDSIDE MANNER QUESTIONS

11. What would your communication style/approach be with this patient?

_____

_____

_____

_____

12. If a patient is distressed by the diagnosis, what might offer support?

_____

_____

_____

_____

ANSWER KEY _available at_
https://connect.springerpub.com/content/book/978-0-8261-8273-9

BACK PAIN AND POOR POSTURE, PEDIATRIC FEMALE

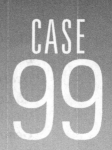

CHIEF COMPLAINT

"Back pain and poor posture."

HISTORY OF PRESENT ILLNESS

A 9-year-old girl is brought to the office by her parents to discuss her poor posture and lingering back pain. They constantly remind her to sit up straight. Their daughter states she tries to sit straight and is doing the best she can. She admits to lingering mid-back pain. The pain is a 4/10, is localized to mid-thoracic area bilaterally, does not migrate, and is described as a consistent ache, not stabbing or pulsatile. The patient takes ibuprofen 200 mg every 6 hours sometimes but usually tries to just ignore her pain. She is not involved in any sports but plays violin and piano. She is active with friends and has not noted any change or limitation in interactions with them. She denies pain in her shoulders or legs. No muscle weakness in her extremities has been noted by her or her parents. They state this has been going on for a while and think they noted the problem the most over the past 6 to 9 months.

REVIEW OF SYSTEMS

The ROS was unremarkable. The girl has mid-thoracic bilateral 4/10 pain as described. The ROS was negative for cough, SOB, chest pain, fatigue, abdominal pain, vomiting, diarrhea, dysuria, fever, muscle weakness, or dizziness.

RELEVANT HISTORY

The patient is fully vaccinated and has had no recent travel; she has no history of prior surgeries or trauma and no chronic health concerns. Her parents recall she reached developmental milestones on time. She has not been to a pediatrician since her kindergarten checkup because her parents' insurance has a high deductible. The child lives with her parents in a house built about 10 years ago. Her parents deny any significant family history of illness.

ALLERGIES

No known food or drug allergies.

MEDICATIONS

Ibuprofen 200 mg q6h PRN for pain.

PHYSICAL EXAMINATION

Vitals: T 37°C (98.6°F); P 80; R 17; BP 116/72; WT 41.27 kg (91 lbs), 90th to 95th percentile; HT 147.32 cm (58 in.), 95th to 100th percentile; BMI 19.

General: Alert and in no distress.

Skin, Hair, and Nails: Warm, dry, with no rashes noted. Capillary refill brisk. No abnormal findings with hair or nails.

Head: Normocephalic and atraumatic.

Neck: Supple with no adenopathy.

Chest: The sternum is normal, with no pectus carinatum or excavatum noted.

Lungs: Clear to auscultation throughout all fields. Aeration is symmetric.

Heart: RRR, with no murmur, gallop, or rub.

Abdomen: Soft, non-tender, non-distended with no masses noted. Bowel sounds equal throughout.

Genital/ Rectal: Tanner stage 1. Rectal exam deferred.

Musculoskeletal: Obvious shoulder height discrepancy with right shoulder elevated. Right scapula is mildly elevated compared to the left. A forward bend test shows noticeable prominence to the right thoracic and ribs in the mid-thoracic range. There is also prominence to the paraspinal muscles of the left lumbar spine. A scoliometer is utilized and shows a 9° angle of rotation over the mid-thoracic spine and 7° angle of rotation over the lumbar spine.

Neurologic: Cranial nerves II to XII intact. DTR symmetric in the upper and lower extremities at 2/4, and muscle strength symmetric in the upper and lower extremities at 5/5.

CLINICAL DISCUSSION QUESTIONS

1. What is the differential diagnosis?

_____

_____

_____

_____

2. What is the most likely diagnosis? Why?

_____

_____

_____

_____

3. Demonstrate your understanding about the pathophysiology in regard to the most likely diagnosis.

_____

_____

_____

_____

4. Should tests/imaging studies be ordered? Which ones? Why? Think about tests/imaging beyond the primary care setting as well.

_____

_____

_____

_____

5. What are the next appropriate steps in management?

_____

_____

_____

_____

6. Discuss screening and treatment recommendations for the diagnosis. Additionally, what role do CM play in the diagnosis? Include references to support your response.

_____

_____

_____

_____

_____

7. What are the pertinent ICD-10 and CPT (E/M) codes for this visit? Provide a short rationale.

_____

_____

_____

_____

_____

8. What is the appropriate patient education topic for this case?

_____

_____

_____

_____

9. If not managed appropriately, what is/are the medical/legal concern(s) that may arise?

_____

_____

_____

_____

10. Think about interprofessional collaboration for this case. Provide a list of specialties or other disciplines and indicate what contribution these professionals might make to managing the patient.

_____

_____

_____

_____

BEDSIDE MANNER QUESTIONS

11. How would you communicate your likely diagnosis to the patient and her parents?

_____

_____

_____

_____

_____

12. If the patient and family show distress at what you communicate, how would you provide support?

_____

_____

_____

_____

_____

ANSWER KEY _available at_
https://connect.springerpub.com/content/book/978-0-8261-8273-9

ITCHY BUMPS, PEDIATRIC FEMALE

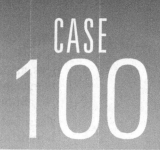

CHIEF COMPLAINT
"Itchy bumps."

HISTORY OF PRESENT ILLNESS
A mother brings her 9-year-old daughter to her PCP for evaluation of an itchy, bumpy rash that comes and goes but resolves within a few hours. This has been going on for 1 month. The last episode of rash was 1 day ago and lasted all day, keeping the child and parent up at night. The rash was accompanied by a swelling of the girl's eyelids. The mother administered diphenhydramine at night, which helped a little. Today, the eye swelling has resolved and the rash is slightly better. The mother was able to take some pictures of the initial rash with her phone. The rash in the pictures shows raised bumps and patches, round or oval across the body, especially on the abdomen, thigh, and back. The patient remembers having a few itchy bumps here and there in the past but thought they were mosquito bites. The patient and mother cannot recall a correlation between rash and possible triggers such as food, contact, or other stressors such as heat, cold, or medications such as NSAIDs. The mother is extremely concerned as she has tried to find answers online and worried her child may have a cancer or leukemia. The mother is unsure of any food allergies.

REVIEW OF SYSTEMS
The patient's ROS is positive for diffuse rash, pruritus, and upper eyelid swelling. Her ROS is negative for unexplained fever, adenopathy, recent unintentional weight loss, fatigue, headache, joint pain or swelling, wheezing, flushing, palpitation, abdominal pain, skin ulceration, wheezing, SOB, and swelling of throat or tongue. She has no history of thyroid dysfunction, vasculitis, or auto-immune-related health problems.

RELEVANT HISTORY
The patient has history of seasonal allergies to pollen and takes loratadine 10 mg daily during spring and early summer. She is up to date on her immunizations. There is no significant contributory history from her family.

ALLERGIES
No known drug allergies; no known food allergies.

MEDICATIONS
Loratadine 10 mg PO daily PRN for seasonal allergies.

PHYSICAL EXAMINATION

Vitals: T 37°C (98.6°F), P 80, R 18, BP 110/72, WT 36.29 kg (80 lbs), HT 142.24 cm (56 in.), BMI 18.

General: A&O, playful, and interactive.

Psychiatry: Normal affect, good eye contact, answers general questions appropriately.

Skin, Hair, and Nails: No lesions or scales in hairline noted. Diffuse raised erythematous and edematous papules and plaques ranging from 0.2 cm to 1 cm present on neck, abdomen, thigh, legs, arm, hands, feet, buttocks, and back. Plantar and palmer surfaces are spared. Lesions are blanchable. No ulceration or target lesion noted. No jaundice noted. Skin has a normal turgor. No abnormal findings with hair or nails.

Eyes: Both eyes with clear sclera and conjunctiva; ophthalmoscope exam shows no sign of hemorrhage.

ENT/Mouth: Both TM clear with cone of light visible; oropharyngeal mucosa without redness or exudate. No swelling of eyelids, lips, or tongue.

Neck: Non-tender, no adenopathy noted.

Lungs: No wheezing, rales, or rhonchi.

Heart: RRR, no murmur noted.

Peripheral Vascular: Good peripheral perfusion present.

CLINICAL DISCUSSION QUESTIONS

1. What is the differential diagnosis?

_____

_____

_____

_____

_____

2. What is the most likely diagnosis? Why?

_____

_____

_____

_____

3. Demonstrate your understanding about the pathophysiology in regard to the most likely diagnosis.

_____

_____

_____

_____

_____

4. Should tests/imaging studies be ordered? Which ones? Why? Think about tests/imaging beyond the primary care setting as well.

_____

_____

_____

_____

5. What are the next appropriate steps in management?

_____

_____

_____

_____

_____

6. What is the diagnostic approach and prognosis for this diagnosis? Provide references for your response.

_____

_____

_____

_____

_____

7. What are the pertinent ICD-10 and CPT (E/M) codes for this visit? Provide a short rationale.

_____

_____

_____

_____

_____

8. What are the appropriate patient/parent education topics for this case?

_____

_____

_____

_____

9. If not managed appropriately, what is/are the medical/legal concern(s) that may arise?

_____

_____

_____

_____

10. Think about interprofessional collaboration for this case. Provide a list of specialties or other disciplines and indicate what contribution these professionals might make to managing the patient.

_____

_____

_____

_____

_____

BEDSIDE MANNER QUESTION

11. What would your communication style/approach be with this parent/patient?

_____

_____

_____

_____

_____

ANSWER KEY _available at_
https://connect.springerpub.com/content/book/978-0-8261-8273-9

FREQUENT ILLNESS AND FATIGUE, ADULT FEMALE

CHIEF COMPLAINT

"Frequent illness and fatigue."

HISTORY OF PRESENT ILLNESS

A 34-year-old African American woman presents for a third time in 6 months complaining of upper respiratory symptoms. At this time, her symptoms, including cough, are resolving. She reports that she tends to get sick easily. She is less concerned about her current symptoms but more concerned about always getting sick. Three months ago, she was also diagnosed with community-acquired pneumonia. Over the past 3 months, she has noted marked fatigue and generalized achiness. Nothing seems to help with her symptoms. She has taken ibuprofen for her symptoms with fair relief. She does not eat a well-balanced diet and calls her diet "the typical American diet."

REVIEW OF SYSTEMS

The patient's ROS is positive for fatigue, generalized myalgias, and a nonproductive resolving cough. She denies recent changes in weight or appetite, heart palpitation, SOB, pale skin (pallor), heat or cold intolerance, nausea, vomiting, diarrhea, constipation, polyuria, polydipsia, polyphagia, headache, dizziness, numbness, and tingling in upper or lower extremities. She also denies fever, chills, and chest pain. She denies anxiety and depression.

RELEVANT HISTORY

Her history is positive for being overweight. She was treated for pneumonia 3 months ago. Her immunizations are up to date. Her surgical history includes a Cesarean section in 2015. She has no hospitalizations outside of childbirth. She was tested for HIV 9 months ago and the result was negative. Her last physical exam was 9 months ago. She has no history of cancer, diabetes, hypertension, or thyroid problems. The patient is married and has two young children. Her marriage is monogamous, and she has been married for 10 years. Her husband had vasectomy a few years ago. She is a kindergarten teacher. She reports missing work at least twice a month due to illness and fatigue. She does not use alcohol, illicit drugs, or tobacco products. She is not physically active and does not spend much time outside. Her family history is non-contributory.

ALLERGIES

Penicillin (hives); no known food allergies.

MEDICATIONS

None.

PHYSICAL EXAMINATION

Vitals: T 36.94°C (98.5°F), P 86, R 16, BP 134/72, WT 68 kg (150 lbs) HT 160 cm (63 in.), BMI 26.6.

General: Well nourished, well developed, in no acute distress. Overweight.

Psychiatric: Calm and cooperative.

Skin, Hair, and Nails: Skin warm and without rash; no pallor of skin; no abnormal findings on hair and nails.

Head: Normocephalic; no deformities noted.

Eyes: PERRLA.

ENT/Mouth: TM clear bilaterally; no pharyngeal erythema; no nasal deformity.

Neck: Supple; no thyromegaly; FROM.

Lungs: Clear to auscultation in all lung fields; no wheezing; no crackles.

Heart: Regular rate and rhythm, no murmurs or gallops noted.

Musculoskeletal: FROM in all extremities; no muscle tenderness with palpation; no edema or deformities noted.

Neurologic: A&O×3; follows commands; cranial nerves II to XII grossly intact.

CLINICAL DISCUSSION QUESTIONS

1. What is the differential diagnosis?

2. What is the most likely diagnosis? Why?

3. Demonstrate your understanding about the pathophysiology in regard to the most likely diagnosis.

4. Should tests/imaging studies be ordered? Which ones? Why? Think about tests/imaging beyond the primary care setting as well.

5. What are the next appropriate steps in management?

_____

_____

_____

_____

6. What are the risk factors and treatment approach of the diagnosis? Provide references for your responses.

_____

_____

_____

_____

7. What are the pertinent ICD-10 and CPT (E/M) codes for this visit? Provide a short rationale.

_____

_____

_____

_____

8. What is the appropriate patient education for this case?

_____

_____

_____

_____

9. If not managed appropriately, what is/are the medical/legal concern(s) that may arise?

_____

_____

_____

_____

10. Think about interprofessional collaboration for this case. Provide a list of specialties or other disciplines and indicate what contribution these professionals might make to managing the patient.

_____

_____

_____

_____

BEDSIDE MANNER QUESTION

11. What would your communication style/approach be with this patient and her parents?

_____

_____

_____

_____

ANSWER KEY *available at*
https://connect.springerpub.com/content/book/978-0-8261-8273-9

LIST OF ABBREVIATIONS

AAFP	American Academy of Family Practice	AMI	Acute myocardial infarction
A1AT	Alpha-1-antitrypsin	ANA	Anti-nuclear antibodies
AAO	Awake, alert, and oriented	ANC	Absolute neutrophil count
AAP	American Academy of Pediatrics	AOM	Acute otitis media
Ab	Antibody	A&O	Alert and oriented
ABG	Arterial blood gas	AP	Advanced placement
ABI	Ankle-brachial index	APC	Adenomatous polyposis coli
ACA	Affordable Care Act	ARBs	Angiotensin receptor blockers
ACE	Angiotensin-converting enzyme	ART	Antiretroviral therapy
ACIP	Advisory Committee on Immunization Practices	ASAP	As soon as possible
		ASCVD	Atherosclerotic cardiovascular disease
ACLE	Acute cutaneous lupus erythematosus	ASD	Autism spectrum disorder
ACLS	Advanced cardiac life support	ASO	Antistreptolysin O
ACS	Acute coronary syndrome	ASQ-3	Ages and Stages Questionnaire, Third Edition
ACTH	Adrenocorticotropic hormone	AST	Aspartate aminotransferase
ADA	Americans with Disabilities Act	AUA	American Urological Association
ADHD	Attention deficit hyperactivity disorder	AUD	Alcohol use disorder
ADLs	Activities of daily living	AUDIT-C	Alcohol Use Disorders Identification Test-Concise
AFP	Alpha-fetoprotein	AV	Atrioventricula
AGEs	Advanced glycation end products	AVL	Augmented vector left
AHI	Apnea-hypopnea index	AVN	Avascular necrosis
AIP	Acute intermittent porphyria	BASE	Brief Abuse Screen of Elderly
AIS	Adolescent idiopathic scoliosis	BG	Blood glucose
AKI	Acute kidney injury	BID	Twice daily
ALP	Alkaline phosphatase	BL	Bilateral
ALT	Alanine transaminase	BLE	Bilateral lower extremity

BMI	Body mass index	CMAP	Compound muscle action potential
BMP	Basic Metabolic Panel	CMP	Comprehensive metabolic panel
BNP	Brain natriuretic peptide	CMV	Cytomegalovirus
BP	Blood pressure	CN	Cranial nerves
BPH	Benign prostatic hypertrophy	CNS	Central nervous system
BRAT	Bananas, rice, applesauce, and toast	COMPLETES	Color, Other conditions, Mobility, Position, Lighting, Entire surface, Translucency, External auditory canal and auricle, Seal
BRCA	Breast cancer gene		
BRUE	Brief resolved unexplained event	COPD	Chronic obstructive pulmonary disease
BS	Bowel sounds		
BUN	Blood urea nitrogen	COVID-19	Coronavirus disease 2019
BV	Bacterial vaginosis	COX	Cyclooxygenase
CAD	Coronary artery disease	CPAP	Continuous positive airway pressure
CBC	Complete blood count		
CBD	Cannabidiol	CPF	Chronic plantar fasciitis
CCBs	Calcium channel blockers	CPS	Child Protective Services
CCM	Chronic care model	CPT	Current Procedural Terminology
CCP	Cyclic citrullinated peptide	CPT (E/M)	Current Procedural Terminology (Evaluation and management)
CD4	Cluster of differentiation 4		
CD8	Cluster of differentiation 8	CRP	C-reactive protein
CDC	Centers for Disease Control and Prevention	CSD	Cat scratch disease
		CSF	Cerebrospinal fluid
CEA	Carcinoembryonic antigen	CTA	Clear to auscultation
CENTOR	Cough, Exudates, Nodes, Temperature, OR	CTS	Carpal tunnel syndrome
		CUP	Cancer of unknown primary
CFS	Cerebrospinal fluid	CV	Cardiovascular
CFU	Colony-forming unit	CVA	Cerebrovascular accident
CGM	Continuous glucose monitor	CVD	Coronary vascular disease
CHF	Congestive heart failure	2D	Two-dimensional
CHIP	Children's Health Insurance Program	DASH	Dietary approaches to stop hypertension
CK	Creatine kinase	DCCT	Diabetes Control and Complications Trial
CKD	Chronic kidney disease		
CKMB	Creatine kinase myocardial band	DDx	Differential diagnosis
CLIA	Clinical Laboratory Improvement Amendments	DEXA	Dual-energy x-ray absorptiometry
		DGP	Deamidated gliadin peptide
CM	Chiari malformations	DJD	Degenerative joint disease

DKA	Diabetic ketoacidosis		EPT	Expedited partner therapy
DM	Diabetes mellitus		ESLD	End-stage liver disease
DMT	Disease-modifying therapy		ESR	Erythrocyte sedimentation rate
DOH	Department of health		ESWT	Extracorporeal shock wave therapy
DSM-5	Diagnostic and Statistical Manual of Mental Disorders, Fifth Edition		FABER	Flexion, abduction, external rotation
DSME	Diabetes self-management, education		FBS	Fasting blood sugar
			FDA	Food and Drug Administration
DSMS	Diabetes self-management, support		FEV1	Forced expiratory volume
DTaP	Diphtheria and tetanus toxoids and acellular pertussis		FM	Fibromyalgia
			FMLA	Family Medical Leave Act
DTR	Deep tendon reflexes		FOBT	Fecal occult blood testing
DVT	Deep vein thrombosis		FODMAP	Fermentable oligosaccharides, disaccharides, monosaccharides and polyols
EB	Elementary body			
EBV	Epstein–Barr virus			
ED	Emergency Department		FPG	Fasting blood glucose
EEG	Electroencephalogram		FQHC	Federally qualified health center
EF	Ejection fraction		FROM	Full range of motion
EGD	Esophagogastroduodenoscopy		FSH	Follicle-stimulating hormone
EGFR	Epidermal growth factor		FSS	Function Status Scale
eGFR	Estimated glomerular filtration rate		FTA-ABS	Fluorescent treponemal antibody absorbed
EHR	Electronic health records		FVC	Forced vital capacity
EIA	Enzyme immunoassay		GP	Gravidity and parity
ELISA	Enzyme-linked immunoassay		GAD	General anxiety disorder
EM	Erythema multiforme		GAD	65 Glutamic acid decarboxylase
EmA	Endomysium antibodies		GAS	Group A streptococcus
EMG	Electromyelography		GBM	Glioblastoma multiforme
EMR	Electronic medical records		GC	Gonococcal
EMS	Emergency medical services		GCA	Giant cell arteritis
EMT	Emergency medical technician		GCS	Glasgow coma scale
ENG	Electronystagmography		GE	Gastroesophageal
ENP	Emergency nurse practitioner		GERD	Gastroesophageal reflux disease
ENT	Ear, nose, throat		GFD	Gluten-free diet
EOM	Extraocular movement		GFR	Glomerular filtration rate
EOMI	Extraocular movements intact		GH	Growth hormone
EP	Electrophysiology		GI	Gastrointestinal

GINA	Global Initiative for Asthma Management and Prevention	IBS	Irritable bowel syndrome
GNAS1	Guanine nucleotide binding protein, alpha stimulating	IBS-C	Irritable bowel syndrome with predominant constipation
GU	Genitourinary	IBS-D	Irritable bowel syndrome with predominant diarrhea
2-h PG	2-hour plasma glucose	ICD	International Classification of Diseases
HAV	hepatitis A virus	IDSA	Infectious Diseases Society of America
HC	Head circumference	IEP	Individualized education program
hCG	Human chorionic gonadotropin	IFA	Immunofluorescent antibody
Hct	Hematocrit	IgA	Immunoglobulin A
HCTZ	Hydrochlorothiazide	IGF-1	Insulin-like growth factor 1
HCV	Hepatitis C virus	IGIM	Intramuscular immunoglobulin
HD	Hypokinetic dysarthria	IgM	Immunoglobulin M
HDL	High-density lipoprotein	IL-15	Interleukin-15
HEENT	Head, Eye, Ear, Nose, and Throat	IM	Intramuscular
HER	Human epidermal growth factor receptor 2	INS	Idiopathic nephrotic syndrome
HF	Heart failure	IOP	Intraocular pressure
HFMD	Hand, foot, and mouth disease	ISD	Intrinsic sphincteric deficiency
Hgb	Hemoglobin	ITP	Idiopathic thrombocytopenic purpura
Hgb A1C	Hemoglobin A1C		
HLA	Human leukocyte antigen	IU	International unit
HNF	Hepatocyte nuclear factor	IUD	Intrauterine device
HPI	History of present illness	IV	Intravenous
HPP	Hypokalemic periodic paralysis	JIA	Juvenile idiopathic arthritis
HPV	Human papillomavirus	JIS	Juvenile idiopathic scoliosis
HR	Heart rate	JRA	Juvenile rheumatoid arthritis
HRA	High-resolution anoscopy	JVD	Jugular Venous Distention
HS	Hidradenitis suppurativa	KRAS	Kirsten rat sarcoma
HSP	Henoch-Schonlein purpura	LABA/ICS	Long-acting beta-agonists and inhaled corticosteroids
HSV	Herpes simplex virus		
HT	Height	LAD	Lymphadenopathy
HTN	Hypertension	LADA	Latent autoimmune diabetes of adulthood
IACS	Intra-articular corticosteroid	LAMA	Long-acting muscarinic antagonist
IBC	Inflammatory breast cancer	LDH	Lactate dehydrogenase
IBD	Inflammatory bowel disease	LDL	Low-density lipoproteins

LES	Lower esophageal sphincter		MRSA	Methicillin-resistant Staphylococcus aureus
LFTs	Liver function tests		MS	Multiple sclerosis
LH	Luteinizing hormone		MSCRAMMs	Microbial surface components recognizing adhesive matrix molecules
LLC	Lower limb cellulitis			
LLQ	Left lower quadrant		MSI	Microsatellite instability
LMP	Last menstrual period		MSM	Men who have sex with men
LP	Lipoprotein		MSSA	Methicillin-sensitive Staphylococcal Aureus
Lp(a)	Lipoprotein(a)			
LPN	Licensed practical nurses		MVA	Motor vehicle accident
LROM	Limited range of motion		NAAT	Nucleic acid amplification test
LS	Lumbar spine		NABS	Normal Active Bowel Sounds
LSM	Lifestyle modifications		NAD	No acute distress
LSW	Licensed clinical social worker		NAFLD	Nonalcoholic fatty liver disease
LVN	Licensed vocational nurse		NASH	Nonalcoholic steatohepatitis
MA	Medical assistant		NCAT	Normocephalic, atraumatic
MALT	Mucosa-associated lymphoid tissue		NCS	Nerve conduction study
MAS	Macrophage activation syndrome		NF	Necrotizing fasciitis
MCH	Mean corpuscular hemoglobin		NGSP	National Glycohemoglobin Standardization Program
MCHC	Corpuscular hemoglobin concentration		NGU	Nongonococcal urethritis
MCLS	Medial collateral ligament strain		NICHQ	National Initiative for Children's Healthcare Quality
MCN	Minimal-change nephropathy			
MCV	Corpuscular volume		NO	Nitric oxide
MD	Meningococcal disease		NOS	Not Otherwise Specified
MDI	Metered dose inhaler		NPO	Nil per os
MDS	Movement Disorder Society		NSAIDs	Nonsteroidal antiinflammatory drugs
MI	Myocardial infarction			
MIRM	Mycoplasma pneumoniae-induced rash and mucositis		NSTEMI	Non-ST segment elevation myocardial infarction
MKPS	Medial knee plica syndrome		NSVD	Normal Spontaneous Vaginal Delivery
MMR	Measles, mumps, and rubella		NTND	Non-tender non-distended
MMRV	Measles, mumps, rubella, and varicella		OA	Osteoarthritis
			OAB	Overactive bladder
MMSE	Mini mental-state exam		OAB-q	Overactive Bladder Questionnaire
MODY	Maturity-onset diabetes of youth		OAB–V8	Overactive bladder-validated 8
MRA	Magnetic resonance angiography		OD	Oculus dexter

ODD	Oppositional defiant disorder	PLT	Platelets
OGTT	Oral glucose tolerance test	PMI	Point of maximal impulse
OM	Otitis media	PMNs	Polymorphonuclear neutrophils
OME	Otitis media with effusion	PNS	Primary nephrotic syndrome
OP	Oropharynx	PO	By mouth
OR	Operating room	POCBG	Point-of-care blood sugar
OS	Oculus sinister (left eye)	POCUS	Point-of-care ultrasound
OSA	Obstructive sleep apnea	PPIs	Proton-pump inhibitors
OT	Occupational Therapy	PR	Plaque rupture
OTC	Over-the-counter	PrEP	Pre-exposure prophylaxis
OU	O´culus uter´que (each eye)	PRN	As needed
PA	Physician assistant	PRP	Platelet-rich plasma
PACE	Program of All-Inclusive Care for the Elderly	PSA	Prostate-specific antigen
PAD	Peripheral arterial disease	PSGN	Post-streptococcal acute glomerulonephritis
PAG	Periaqueductal gray matter	PT	Physical therapist
PBP-2a	Penicillin-binding protein 2A	PTA	Peritonsillar abscess
PCOS	Polycystic ovarian syndrome	PTH	Parathyroid hormone
PCP	Primary care physician	PTNS	Peripheral tibial nerve stimulation
PCR	Polymerase chain reaction	PTT	Partial thromboplastin time
PCV13	Pneumococcal conjugate vaccine 13	PVCs	Premature ventricular contractions
PD	Parkinson's disease	QD	Daily
PE	Pulmonary embolism	QHS	Every night at bedtime
PERRL	Pupil, equal, round, reactive (to), light	QID	Four times daily
		QTC	QT interval corrected
PERRLA	Pupil, equal, round, reactive (to), light, accommodation	RAAS	Renin–angiotensin–aldosterone system
PF	Plantar flexion	RAI	Radioactive iodine therapy
PFS	Patellofemoral syndrome	RAMs	Rapid alternating movements
PHQ	Personal health questionnaire	RB	Reticulate body
PHQ-9	Personal Health Questionnaire-9	RBC	Red blood cell
PI	Phosphatidylinositol	RBS	Random blood sugar
PICU	Pediatric ICU	RDW	Red cell distribution width
PID	Pelvic inflammatory disease	RF	Rheumatoid factor
PKC	Protein kinase C	RICE	Rest, ice, compression, and elevation
PKD	Polycystic kidney disease	RIDT	Rapid Influenza Diagnostic Test

RLQ	Right lower quadrant	SSS	Symptom Severity Scale
RMSF	Rocky Mountain spotted fever	SSTI	Skin and soft tissue infection
ROM	Range of motion	STAT	Immediately
ROS	Review of systems	STDs	Sexually transmitted diseases
RPR	Rapid plasma reagin	STEMI	ST-segment elevation myocardial infarction
RR	Regular rate	STI	Sexually transmitted infection
RRMS	Relapsing remitting multiple sclerosis	T1DM	Type 1 diabetes mellitus
RRR	Regular rate and rhythm	T2DM	Type 2 diabetes mellitus
RSR	Regular sinus rhythm	TAH/BSO	Total Abdominal Hysterectomy with Bilateral Salpingo-Oophorectomy
RSV	Respiratory Syncytial Virus	TB	Tuberculosis
RT-PCR	Reverse transcription polymerase chain reaction	TBI	Traumatic brain injury
RUQ	Right upper quadrant	Tdap	Tetanus, diphtheria, acellular pertussis
RZV	Recombinant zoster vaccine	TEACCH	Treatment and Education of Autistic and related Communication Handicapped
SA	Sinoatrial	TG	Transglutaminase
SB	Sickle beta	THC	Tetrahydrocannabinol
SC	Sickle cell	TIBC	Total iron binding capacity
SCC	Staphylococcal chromosome cassette	TID	Three times a day
SCD	Sickle cell disease	TM	Tympanic membrane
SCQ	Social Communication Questionnaire	TMN	Thin membrane nephropathy
SG	Specific gravity	TMP–SMX	Trimethoprim–sulfamethoxazole
SHBG	Sex hormone binding globulin	TPO	Thyroid peroxidase
SIRS	Systemic inflammatory response syndrome	TPP	Thyrotoxic periodic paralysis
SJIA	Systemic juvenile idiopathic arthritis	TRT	Testosterone replacement therapy
SJS	Steven-Johnson Syndrome	TSH	Thyroid-stimulating hormone
SLE	Systemic lupus erythematosus	TSH-R	Thyroid-stimulating hormone
SLR	Straight leg raise	TSI	Thyroid-stimulating immunoglobulin
SOAP	Subjective, objective, assessment, and plan	TTG	Tissue transglutaminase
SOB	Shortness of breath	TTP	Thrombotic thrombocytopenic purpura
SRCs	Sports-related concussions	TV	Trichomonas vaginalis
SSRIs	Selective serotonin reuptake inhibitors	UA	Urine analysis
		UAhCG	Urine analysis human chorionic gonadotropin

UC	Ulcerative colitis	UVB	Ultraviolet B
UE	Upper extremity	VDRL	Venereal Disease Research Laboratory
URI	Upper respiratory infection	WBC	White blood cell
US	Ultrasound	WHO	World Health Organization
USPSTF	United States Preventive Services Task Force	WNL	Within normal limit
UTI	Urinary tract infection	WT	Weight
UV	Ultraviolet		

Printed in the United States
by Baker & Taylor Publisher Services